Oars for Pleasure Rowing

Their Design and Use

by
Andrew B. Steever

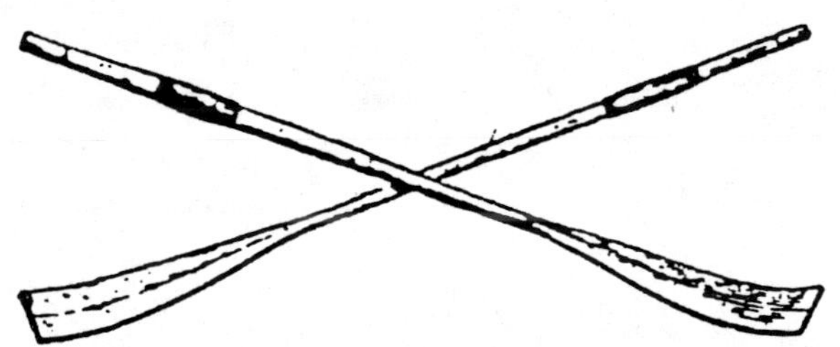

Mystic Seaport Museum, Inc.
Mystic, Connecticut
1993

Oars for Pleasure Rowing

The major portions of this work, published in *Lines & Offsets* 35-40 (December 1982-November 1983), are reprinted with the permission of Robert B. Chapel.

ISBN 0-913372-65-X

"...and just then a wager-boat flashed into view, the rower, a short, stout figure, splashing badly and rolling a good deal, but working his hardest. The Rat stood up and hailed him, but Toad - for it was he - shook his head and settled sternly to his work."

Kenneth Grahame
The Wind in the Willows

CONTENTS

FOREWORD

Rowing as a means of moving boats on the water began so far back in time that no remembrance of when remains; yet rowing for enjoyment - rowing for the sheer pleasure of rowing - is something quite new. For centuries rowing was work-tedious, taxing exertion to be avoided when possible, and becoming in the row galleys of the ancient world, punishment for criminals and the unhappy fate of thousands of unfortunate slaves chained to their oars.

With the coming of the outboard motor and it's wide-spread distribution, rowing in this country nearly died out, that is with the exception of the special case of competitive rowing in racing shells, a narrowly restricted collegiate sport. Fifteen years ago it appeared that most people not only no longer rowed, or had any need to, but had forgotten how. Then at deepest ebb the tide turned, and today, scarcely more than a decade later, people in increasing numbers are rowing once again, and for the enjoyment of it. At one gathering this summer, for a cross-Sound row in Washington, boats numbered nearly 300, I have been told, with more than 400 rowers pulling at the oars.

How to account for this rowing resurgence? There are a variety of contributing factors, of course. But certainly high on the list is the enthusiasm and expertise of rowing buffs such as Andy Steever. Steever's love affair with rowing began years ago when as a small boy he discovered the joys of pleasure rowing in a St. Lawrence River skiff, amidst the scenic delights of the Thousand Islands.

In this treatise on "Oars For Pleasure Rowing" two Steevers are in evidence; one, the rowing enthusiast who delights in rowing for the sheer, uncomplicated physical pleasure of

doing it; the other, the scientist and engineer who applies his investigative tools and methodology to the pleasure oar as he would to a machine, in order to analyze and quantify it's mechanical operation. And it is here that Steever makes his special, and in fact, his unique contribution. Here for the first time anywhere, I believe, is to be found a technical explanation of the mechanical principles of pleasure oar design. Anyone can immediately feel the world of difference between properly shaped and balanced oars for recreational rowing, and those heavy, clumsy slabs of timber that so frequently pass for oars, turning many against rowing for the rest of their lives. But it is quite a different thing to understand the mechanical principles that make oars superior, and only as these are understood and applied may we expect any widespread improvement in oars such as are now used.

Those whose strengths are not in math and physics may find following Steever in some of his technical explanations hard going. Never mind, there is plenty for them too. How to balance and tune oars for easy, efficient performance; how to trim and shave them to correct proportions; wider tips for greater effectiveness; two pairs of oars, one a shorter, easier-pulling pair, for up-wind work, the other, a harder pulling pair, longer with wider tips, for faster, calm, or downwind pulling; locks, their selection and care; stretchers, fitting them and the boat to the oarsman - all of this and much more is clearly and fully set forth.

Some may find Steever's focus narrow in it's restriction to an analysis of the kind of rowing Steever knows best and is personally most interested in, namely rowing on the gunwale "in <u>fixed-seat</u> rowboats, one hand per oar," or scull, as oars so used are called. To have enlarged his investigations to include sliding-seat rowing, after the manner of the racing shell, would have required a much more

extensive effort than the one reported here. Nevertheless, Steever has laid the groundwork for such an effort, established principles and set up parameters for a scientific investigation of sliding-seat pleasure rowing when such is undertaken.

One final thing to be mentioned here: it becomes clear in reading Steever's account that there is much interesting fun to be had with a pair of oars before they are in the boat and rowing. To design, or work over the design of a pair of oars, shaving and shaping them, balancing and tuning them, can be an intensely interesting and pleasurable experience in itself. Quite possibly the ultimate in rowing pleasure is not possible until one is rowing with a pair of oars that he conceived and crafted, balanced and tuned, himself.

John Gardner

PREFACE

Oars are a dandy subject with lots of traditional flavor stemming from ancient customs and hard usage. But are old customs relevant to modern pleasure rowing in recreational boats? The object of this study is the analysis of pleasure oar design for fixed seat row boats, one hand per oar. It includes comments on the physical reasons for certain oar usages and on tuning oars for better performance.

The reader who seeks a simple rule with which to choose an oar will conclude there isn't one which effectively matches the oar and oarsman to his boat, wind, and water. In practice these things are usually changing. However, an analysis of oars and their action may be useful to oar designers, makers, users, and experimenters. Many challenges lie in a wooden stick. I have tried to show, with original research, a fairly rational method of designing and selecting oars. There is little here on making oars after they are designed. For this refer to R.D. Culler's excellent book, Boats, Oars, and Rowing.

Oars for performance inevitably attract Physics and Mathematics. I have kept the math simple and supplemented it with physical descriptions for better reader understanding.

As artifacts, oars have logical features for pleasure rowing as distinct from work boat or racing shell rowing, although there are things to be learned from both ends of the oar spectrum. A good pleasure oar generally feels lighter and requires more care than a fisherman's oar. It will usually be used by a less rugged rower than the racer or fisherman, and in a boat with a potential speed between the two. High efficiency and easy operation are important because fun is the object.

Let's define pleasure rowing as the easiest way for recreational oarsmen to move a responsive boat which is likely to encounter a wide variety of weather on different occasions. Perhaps one day a short leisurely jaunt is just right. Another time it may be an all day row of many scenic miles in weather ranging from a hot calm to an exhilarating pace in rough open water. Or if the boat is a fast one, a bit of racing sport just for the fun of it. All this pleasure rowing depends on the rower's physical condition, temperament, and mood of the moment.

Acknowledgements. I am indebted to Mr. and Mrs. Howard Seaman for permission to mention their fine Adirondack guide-boat oars and also, along with Mr. Fred Burns, for the all-too-short opportunities to watch and photograph guide boats in action and to talk about and row them. I am also indebted to Mr. John Gardner, as many others of us are on a multitude of small craft matters, for his help and encouragement, and the opportunity to include some Mystic Seaport oars. And I warmly appreciate his fine introduction, written at the suggestion of Mr. Robert Chapel. My deep thanks go to Mr. Chapel for his excellent editing and his willingness to include this serial article in his Lines and Offsets. Without him, this work probably wouldn't have appeared. There are a great number of others to whom I am thankful for conversations, correspondence, and reading about oars. Surely none of the above will agree with everything set forth here, so any mistakes are mine. The buck starts and stops here on the "backyard physics" of the characteristic oar numbers. And, of course, I am most indebted to the fabulous St. Lawrence River and its skiffs. Finally, I warmly thank Mystic Seaport Museum, Messrs. Ben Fuller, Gerald Morris, and Andrew German and staff, for this fine revival of the Lines and Offsets articles.

{1}
The Human Engine

This contraption is so feeble that it depends on persistence and continuous coaching by a brain to make a rowboat go. It also has a bio-mechanical memory for repetitive motion and can get set in it's ways unless faced with new situations. It's power output ranges from about 1/15 horsepower for perhaps a day, up to about 1/2 h.p. for two hours for an oarsman in superb condition, until he is temporarily burned out. This puny power level needs ingenuity to direct it efficiently, and the thinking starts with the designs for the oars and boat. This human "prime mover" is highly adaptable, having coped over ages with a vast array of good and bad oars, boats, and weather. So oar features evolved differently in various parts of the world; furthermore what is sacred in one place is disdained in another.

For pleasure rowing this "engine" doesn't like the extremes of a very hard, slow, or short pull or a too easy, fast, or long pull. The "engine's" joints, muscles, and tendons object to the former and the internal friction and inertia of the parts waste too much energy for the latter. However, there is no universally optimum stroke rate for pleasure rowing. Most of us seem to row comfortably and efficiently around 25 to 30 strokes per minute (spm). We can adapt ourselves to as low as 15 spm and temporarily go up to 55 spm with non-feathering oars (somewhat less for feathering) to gain some immediate objective. During a day's row the oarsman may cover this whole range.

There is a certain amount of "tow-rope" energy needed to move a given loaded boat a given distance in a given time in a calm on still water. However, the energy burned by the rower is three to four times greater because neither his

nor the oar's efficiency is 100%. If we can find ways to make the oars more efficient, use them more efficiently, and get the engine tuned up, then the rower will have a wider choice of action. He will reach his destination on less energy, get there sooner, or - possibly of greater interest - row farther on the same amount of energy. Since the "tow-rope" energy needed to go a given distance varies as the second to third power of speed, a rower has a wide choice of gait according to his stamina, available time, and efficiency level.

Pleasure rowing is enhanced by the rower's good condition and vice versa. If the pleasure is also in fabulous surroundings stretching as far as the eye can see, what more can one ask? It is also important to be in good shape for windward and high spirited rowing, which can be great fun.

{2}
Basic Oar Properties

Basic properties of oars are listed in the sections that follow. Many of us have attended rowboat regattas that have sprung up during the last two decades. Noticeable is the great difference in the "feel" of untuned oars when comparing various boats and their rowing equipment. Thus this study. Here the "feel" of oars is described by numbers rather than by subjective impressions.

{3}

Balance

An oar is balanced when held horizontally in it's lock by the limp weight of the rower's hand and forearm on the grip, with the blade motionless out of water. So three balance conditions are needed: a particular person and a particular oar with a particular pivot. Of course this means an oar should be custom fitted to each rower and lock, and right away precludes most standard oars made by rote, such as mass produced unbalanced commercial oars without buttons. However, after purchase many such oars can be custom fitted to an individual by added work. Each oar needs a force P (pounds) downward on the grip to balance it. (Note the balance diagram on Table 1 in the appendix, which lists a few of the oars I have measured over the last 12 years). The P of these oars is shown in column 14. For comparison, a rower can find his own P by resting his hand on the kitchen scales.

Unless an oar is purposely counterbalanced, it's P usually exceeds the rower's P and the oar feels blade-heavy. This is true of most hardwood and the longer softwood oars. A simple balance test can be made outside the boat by horizontally resting the oar at it's lock position on the edge of one's left hand, putting the right hand on the grip. If the right hand is limp, the oar is balanced. Rarely is a balanced oar encountered. But when it is, the owner enjoys one of the secrets of easy rowing because none of his meager energy wastefully bears down on the grip. Unbalanced traditional oars were used by rugged working folk who got used to unbalance at an early age. But for many lightly built folks whose rowing is a sometime thing, the traditional oars seem blade heavy and unwieldy.

The fact that blade buoyancy reduces the oar's P is not

significant, since this happens on the pulling stroke (more about this later). Also, a good blade should be as thin as possible, which minimizes buoyancy. An oar's P can be measured by either of two ways: First, support the oar horizontally at it's center of gravity (c.g) on a scale and apply the leverage principle: P=MxC/(B-2"), where M in pounds is oar weight; C in inches is distance from c.g. to lock center; B in inches is distance from lock to oar end at grip; and 2" corrects B to bring P to mid-grip. This method also yields oar weight and location of c.g., which are used later to determine oar inertia.

The second method finds P directly by supporting the oar horizontally at its lock and hanging an adjusted weight, P, pounds, at 2" from the grip end until the oar balances.

Note that the unbuttoned feathering oar which can slide to and fro in the lock has no definite lock location, hence no unique P value. Some folks might find a place along the leather where the oar balances for them and incidentally produces a certain overlap, if any, of the grips. But whether a lubricated unbuttoned feathering oar will stay put at that balance point on the lock is questionable. Maybe a few fortunate folks can keep it there but many cannot. An oar without a definite lock pivot is unfinished for many pleasure rowers. In this respect a good feathering pleasure oar is like a racing spoon oar which invariably has a button, and such a pleasure oar differs from the usual buttonless fisherman's oar. Most non-feathering oars in this country have definite pivots.

It is sometimes stated that the c.g. of an oar should lie just outside the lock or beyond the leather. This is vague advice as it depends on how far "just outside" is, the oar's weight, the rower's build, and the leather's length.

Blade-heavy oars can be improved as follows: First, thin the blade to the desired spring (more on spring later), if it is not already a cupped blade that may crack if spring is imparted to it. However, some cupped spoons can be thinned without giving them spring. If possible without weakening the oar, and if there is more than enough blade area, gradually remove blade area at the inner end, (more about this later). For a straight-bladed oar try to make the working face flat or slightly concave, with the crown for strength on the forward face. This may make the oars permanently right and left handed. The blade is the most effective place to remove weight because it is farthest from the lock. Second, shave the outer loom until it has the desired spring, bearing in mind that the bending moment and therefore the loom cross-section increases while approaching the lock. The cross-section should be greater fore and aft than vertically in order to withstand the pull. An oval cross-section is fine. However, for the very limber oar for a light boat with non-feathering oars, such as the Adirondack guide boat, the outer loom near the neck has the oval cross-section with the short axis in the direction of the pull and the long axis is vertical to give more stiffness vertically. It would not do to make the short axis vertical. That would make the oar more limber vertically than horizontally. See Pleasure Oar Improvements (section 17) for comments on the guide-boat oar. Some springiness in the blade and outer loom is a good sign that the wood is stressed and "pulls it's weight." However, the wood must be free of defects in order to impart it's maximum strength. Third, using kitchen scales (an indispensable oarmaking and tuning tool) add counterweight close to the grip. Sometimes extra wood left with a square or rectangular section on the inner loom is enough. But if more weight is needed, add lead near or within the grip if it is large enough. The amount of lead is found by balancing the oar at the lock with a hand on the grip and

taping pieces of lead to the loom near the grip until the P of the rower and oar match. Then try the oars in the boat. When satisfactory, form the lead into a slug let into the loom, or use lead shot. Solid lead occupies 2.43 cu. in./lb., while lead shot needs about 3.7 cu. in./lb. For a feathering oar the slug's c.g. should be on the centerline of the oar so there will be no unbalanced rolling torque.

There is less tendency to blister the hand with a balanced oar since the hand only bears it's own weight on the grip. This is particularly helpful to some pleasure rowers whose hands may be soft, and for distance rowers.

It is unlikely that enough balancing lead would be added to sink an oar if it got overboard, but I once checked after adding two pounds. The oar floated level.

If two different pairs of oars are taken on a long row, one pair balanced, the other definitely blade heavy, and the heavy oars are rowed steadily for several hours, one's reflexes so automatically bear down on the grips during the recovery that a peculiar sensation occurs if a quick change is made to the balanced oars. Unconsciously, the hands bear down on the grips as before. Consequently the blades pop high out of the water on the recovery and the rower just can't keep them low until his system adjusts to the new situation. Using the same oars in reverse sequence, the rower can't get the heavy blade out of the water without extra exertion. This experience, in addition to showing the conditioned reflexes of the "human engine" resulting from extended practice, emphasizes the advantage of balanced oars for long rows. Something like this balance sensation may happen when a rower accustomed to heavy oars all his life finds himself in a different boat with balanced oars for the first time. He has to re-learn to row, keeping the blades down on the recovery stroke. For more on taking two

different pairs of oars on long rows later, see <u>Slip</u> (section 6).

Non-feathering oars can be counterweighted so their P equals the rower's P. But the blades of feathering oars, when partially feathered in a strong head wind, tend to lift a little so there may be a reason for some rowers to not fully counterweight feathering oars, particularly if the oars might be used by someone of heavier build than the owner.

Oars 9A, 12A, and 24A in Table 1 are good candidates for tuning. Oar 24A is an interesting one included here because, if it is rowed at the button, it's short inner loom exaggerates it's properties. It is used in a boat with only 39-1/2" beam outside the planking with the locks on the rail. Keep this commercial oar in mind as the rest of this tale unfolds. It's redeeming feature is the moderately short spoon blade.

Before continuing, a few words are in order on my rationale for the limited selection of oars and boats in Table 1. Lack of space prevents more entries. The oars were chosen to show tuned compared to untuned oars, the latter being recognizable by stiffness and much imbalance. I sought also to illustrate the various oar characteristics. The boat types are all easy-running fixed-seat craft that happen to be among the lighter and narrower traditional craft. The Herreshoff/Gardner boat was first built by John Gardner from his interpretation of L. Francis Herreshoff's rough sketch. The detailed construction plans were published in <u>National Fisherman</u>, February-May 1980. I believe the reasons this boat moves so easily are that it has only about 25 sq. ft. of wetted surface on a waterline of 15'-11" with a 165 lb. oarsman, and its displacement curve is sharper at the ends than for most boats. With one rower,

the displacement is about 300 lbs. Several have already been built, and I hope there will be more to come as it is a very good pleasure boat.

{4}

Oar Inertia

While the P of an oar is the static vertical force downward on the grip to balance it out of water, there is also a periodic dynamic horizontal force F, lbs., on the grip due to the inertia and angular acceleration of the oar as it moves to and fro. F is shown in column 17 of Table 1 and the accompanying inertia diagram. This inertia force is separate from the power pull.

Once an oar is swinging at a constant angular velocity about a vertical axis through the lock, its angular acceleration is zero, and its horizontal inertia force on the grip is also zero. It is this way near mid-stroke. However, at both ends of the stroke, the swinging direction is suddenly reversed, causing angular acceleration and then the inertia of the oar is felt as F, lbs., at the grip. Call this angular acceleration, a, radians per second squared (1 radian equals 57.4 degrees of arc). So to have a force F, there must be both an intrinsic inertia property, I, of the oar, and a motion characteristic of angular acceleration, a. F is unimportant for a short, light oar, or if the stroke rate is low. But F is noticeable otherwise principally at both ends of the stroke.

While the above describes physically what occurs, the concise terms of mechanics show F=axI/(B-2"). Where F and a are as above, I is moment of inertia of the oar about a vertical swinging axis at the lock, lbs. x inches x seconds squared. (B-2") is the familiar lever arm, inches, from grip center to lock. It is seen that longer inner looms tend to reduce F. I is measured by hanging the oar on a knife edge clamped to the blade tip, swinging it as a compound pendulum, and counting the number of swings (to and fro equals one swing) in say two minutes to find the

period of the oar, T, seconds per swing. Then knowing the weight of the oar and location of c.g. (from the balance tests), I is calculated from the expressions shown in Table 1. The measurement of angular acceleration, a, requires test equipment. For our purposes, a can be approximated mathematically if harmonic motion of the grip to and fro is assumed. This analysis is omitted here but the result is (a/8)=(t/40) squared, where t is the number of pulling strokes per minute and a is the angular acceleration at the stroke ends.

For example, oar 8B in Table 1 has an I of 8.7. If it is rowed at 40 pulls/minute, it will have an approximate F of 3.3 lbs. at the stroke ends. Oar 31B at 25 pulls/minute will have an F of 2 lbs.

It might be thought that F is too small in comparison with the power pull on the grips. However, F occurs as a push against the hand (or its callouses) at the beginning of the recovery and as an added pull on the hand at the beginning of the pulling stroke. So F may occur 500 to 800 times per mile. Or in a nice 20 mile row, F is applied 10,000 to 16,000 times. How small must F be to be insignificant when applied that many times?

Adding counterweights to balance an oar will increase F. But this is a good trade-off since the counterweights help all the time and F comes mainly at the ends of the stroke and at the higher stroke rates. The advantages of a light blade and outer loom appear three ways: there is less oar to carry (important for Adirondack guide boats), less counterweight to balance the oar, and less oar inertia with a more responsive oar.

There is a practical limit to thinning a wooden blade if it must tangle with lobster pot buoys, rocks, stumps, flotsam,

other oars in a race, etc. Though objectionable to traditionalists, some of the newer materials alone or in combination with wood, result in more durable and lighter blades. This trend exists in canoe and kayak paddles, the design of which is usually more technically advanced than that of most pleasure oars. One reason is that the paddler has to hold up the entire weight of his paddle, while the locks support the oars' weight.

{5}

Oar Stiffness

Among racing shell oarsmen, this is a debatable subject because there is a delayed application of energy to the blade at the beginning of the pull due to energy absorbed by the spring of the oar and a release of this energy at the end of the pull. This affects the oarsman's timing. However, those fellows put more energy in a stroke. For pleasure oars in fixed seat boats that are going at less than maximum speed most of the time, it is hard to see that this energy transfer is that important. In addition to the lighter weight advantage of a limber oar, spring reduces the shock loading on the rower's own "machinery" when the pull is applied. This is beneficial on the long rows and with harder pulling oars. Some canoeists like limber paddles for the same reason. However, a very limber oar has to be used cautiously, and so some owners are careful to whom they loan their choice oars. Many an oar has snapped on a strong, careless, or intentional yank, since water is then about as solid as concrete. Ash and soft maple (which isn't very soft) have good shock resistance, but spruce is only moderately resistant.

Table 1, columns 18 and 19, show some measured spring values made according to the accompanying spring test diagram. For more on stiffness see Very Limber Oars (section 24).

{6}

Slip

One nice thing about oars is that they dip into a medium that won't stay put, and this blessing reduces the shock load of the pull on the rower. So all oars have more or less slip, defined here as the relative velocity of some point on the blade with respect to undisturbed water. Since a point on an oar travels in a circular arc with respect to the lock, the slip at the tip is usually greater than elsewhere for a normal pull.

The blade exerts force on the water only because there is slip. The force depends approximately on the square of the slip velocity, the blade area, and some blade shape coefficient. Thus a modest increase in slip velocity results in substantial increase in blade force. This observation leads to two others: First, since slip is greatest at the tip, a square inch of tip area has more force on it than a square inch elsewhere. Second, high slip oars which have narrow blades must be long enough to slow the stroke rate to within the rower's best range of physical efficiency. And likewise, short oars must reduce slip with wider blades to also slow the stroke rate. However, slip also depends on how fast the boat is running due to its design, loading, wind and wave conditions, and rowing effort.

Before tackling the details of slip a few more observations should be made. The long narrow coastal blade of history has descended to us for several reasons. It is easier and quicker to shape out of stock, and there is less wood wastage than for a wide bladed oar. In former times the production of oars was much greater than at present and more narrow bladed oars could be gotten out of a given butt log of oar-quality wood. For heavy usage in fishing and

working craft, a narrow blade is more durable than a wide one unless the latter has a thicker blade, which would make it blade heavy. Also, the higher freeboard of coastal fishing boats and ancient ships needed longer oars to reach the water. However, these old conditions apply less to the present-day pleasure rowboat. There is no doubt that the inner end of a long blade has less drive. Early racing shell oars had long spoon blades, but modern racing blades are shorter and wider, concentrating area nearer the tip. This idea of wider and shorter blades can be applied to flat-bladed pleasure oars, resulting in improved propulsion efficiency as will be shown later.

Narrow, easily moved, low-freeboard inland rowboats such as the Adirondack guide boat and the St. Lawrence skiff get into narrow water so their oars must be short, and short oars stow better. To do this the blades must be wider with less slip, and wide lumber was available for these boats' oars.

Thus, within the limits of oar dimensions imposed by structural materials there are infinite combinations of oar and blade lengths, blade width and shape, and slip for a given stroke rate and boat speed. However, some combinations have better propulsive efficiency. But due to the ways local customs have grown, each kind of oar has its own advocates who claim no other oar will do.

A way to rationalize the action of different oar types and show the effect of slip is with velocity vector diagrams, figures 1a through 1h for a flat blade (see appendix for all figures). Analogous diagrams are used to analyze velocities in bladed rotating machinery such as pumps, turbines, propellers, etc. So why not apply the idea to one of mankind's earliest bladed tools, the oar? For readers unfamiliar with vectors, these slip diagrams are not hard

to fathom and they yield much information. Just remember in the following that a velocity vector is simply an arrow on paper that has two properties; direction and length proportional to speed. So drawing vectors to scale in the proper direction provides a clear, easy, graphic way of finding the resultant velocity of several simultaneous velocities existing at a point.

The two velocities to be combined are the tangential oar velocity, U, at some point on the oar with respect to the oar lock, and the speed V, of the boat (oarlock) through the water in order to find a resulting slip velocity S, of that point on the blade with respect to the undisturbed water. All velocities are shown in feet/second and are drawn to the same scale (1 knot is 1.69 feet/second).

Figure 1a shows just the U velocities of a blade when the oar is assumed to turn at an angular velocity m, of 1.8 radians per second (equivalent to 103 degrees/second) and when the oar is passing through its thwartwise position. The greatest tangential velocity of 10 feet/second is at the tip and it decreases linearly back along the blade and outer loom to the lock.

Figure 1b indicates the oar when it is momentarily thwartwise with just the boat velocity V, ahead through the water assumed at 3-1/2 knots shown uniformly at all points along the oar. Figure 1c vectorially adds the oar and boat velocities together to give the resultant slip velocity S at the various points along the blade. Note that the slip is greatest at the tip and diminishes to zero farther inboard at some point A where the oar and boat velocities are equal but in opposite directions. Point A can be called a "water pivot."

Since the oar also has a mechanical lock pivot with respect

to the boat, let's keep these two pivots separate ideas even though they are related. Also note that if any part of the oar is immersed inboard of Point A it will have a negative slip and will push water ahead at the expense of lost energy. Negative slip can be seen sometimes with too long a blade or when the oar is immersed so deeply that the loom enters the water too near the boat. Some beginners are apt to row this way. If the distance between the lock and Point A is denoted by r, inches, then r=12 V/m. Note in this example that the blade near the neck has only 1/40th of the slip at the tip, so the water force per sq. in. of blade at the neck end is only 1/1600th of that at the tip. Thus a considerable amount of blade at its inner end, though not as bad as next to the neck, produces less blade force than at the tip, but still it has windage and weight. This shows the benefit of less inner end blade area if Point A is near the neck.

If figure 1c is repeated, but the boat speed V is increased 25% to 7.4 feet/second (the same boat is lighter or there is a wind aft), but the stroke rate and length is unchanged, then figure 1d is obtained, showing that Point A has moved outward and now the blade inner end is pushing water ahead and the blade from Point A to the tip has less slip than before in figure 1c. Consequently the blade now exerts less force on the water and on the rower. Thus the same oar has become <u>easier</u> pulling, which experience says actually happens. To avoid the lost energy due to negative blade slip inboard of Point A, if it is a continuing problem, pare off the blade inboard of Point A if there is enough oar strength left to do so.

Another slip example would be starting again with figure 1c, but adding a strong headwind to slow the boat's forward velocity to one half. But if the oar velocity U, is kept the same as in figure 1a then figure 1e shows the resulting

slip velocity S, has increased over figure 1c. Consequently this will cause a harder pull on the same oar, which again corresponds with experience. The difference between easy and hard pulling on the same oar is felt when quickly turning a boat 180 degrees into a strong wind.

So these slip diagrams are leading to the concepts of easy and hard pulling oars. Unfortunately, there is no simple way to accurately design an oar for just the right pull intensity, since it depends on boat speed, the rower's strength, and the use. If the conditions are such that an oar has too hard a pull, the stroke rate will drop and the oar will tend to pull the rower's arms out of his sockets. So a basically hard pulling oar should be used when the boat is running easily at which time the oar will have a more normal feeling to its pull. Likewise an easier pulling oar should be used when the boat is not running easily.

As an example for all-day rowing when various wind and water conditions are likely to affect boat speed, I carry two different pairs of nicely balanced limber oars. One pair is easy pulling, 7'-8" long with 6-3/8" wide tips for slow going against a strong wind or with a heavy load, or in tight channels. The other pair has a hard pull, 9' long with 7" tip width and is used when the boat wants to run easily in a light headwind or when lightly loaded, and for joy rides down strong winds. These are oars 43A and 31B in Table 1. Some folks laugh when they see those big elephant ears flapping, but they sure can move the boat. The more responsive the boat speed, the more helpful it is to carry two different pairs of oars.

These slip diagrams can explain some other conditions. For example, if the stern painter happens to be still tied to the dock when blithely off we go with zero boat velocity, Figure 1a shows that all the oar velocity is also slip.

This would be the time the oars pull hardest. And it also approximates the situation when getting under way with the first stroke in a heavy boat that hasn't really started to move. Also note that the "water pivot" has moved inboard to the lock.

Another situation shows up in figure 1f, where the boat velocity exceeds the oar tip speed. Here all oar slip is negative, the oar backs water, and Point A is theoretically beyond the tip.

These diagrams show how Point A moves in and out along the oar according to how fast the boat and oars move. Point A is only noticeable (sometimes it is in the water, sometimes above the water in the outer loom) when the oar is thwartwise, and here Point A is the exact distance from the lock, r=12V/m.

When the oar is not thwartwise Point A doesn't exist and then slip always has a lateral component. Figure 1g shows the oar in the first part of the stroke. The resultant slip velocity S, is oblique to the blade and at the tip is pushing some water outward from the boat. The intensity and angle to the blade of this oblique slip changes along the blade length and changes with the angular oar position. Even though this motion in both fore and after strokes is very complicated, some conclusions can be drawn. As water flows obliquely along the blade length some of it spills over the long blade edges. A sharply raised ridge down the blade center, sometimes seen on very handsome oars, will promote this spill-over, which increases slip and ineffiency. Also the long narrow blade will unfavorably spill relatively more obliquely flowing water over its long edges than a short wider blade.

A further advantage of the wider blade shows up in the fore

stroke with the water that approaches the tip edge. More water is kicked aft. This effect is enhanced by curving the end of the oar into a spoon blade to reduce the shock loss of the water obliquely entering the tip edge.

Figure 1h shows slip velocities for a typical oar position aft of thwartwise. Here the oblique slip velocities are inward toward the boat, just the reverse of the fore stroke. Again the same conclusions can be drawn that a wide blade should be more efficient than a narrow one and there should be no blade center ridge.

The spoon oar, due to its tip angle, works better in the fore stroke than in the after stroke. This will be covered in <u>Blade Area and Shape</u> (section 15), and figure 5.

A flat-bladed oar when thwartwise will have some water spilling outward over the tip edge. The blade would be more efficient and have less slip if this endwise spill did not exist. The curved tip of a spoon oar does inhibit endwise spill-over and slip to some extent, thus increasing the blade efficiency when the oar is thwartwise.

The inner blade ends of figures 1g and 1h show the slip velocities are nearly along the blade. Since these velocities are lower and the blade area there relatively small, the inner blade ends don't do much work.

The cure for the ineffective inner blade ends in figures 1g and 1h is to shorten the blades at their inner ends if possible and keep the stroke short. Also note the figures 1c, 1g, and 1h all have the same oar and boat velocities. Therefore the poor behavior at the inner blade end in figures 1g and 1h can be inferred from figure 1c where Point A can be easily seen at mid-stroke to be too close to the blade inner end. The inner blade end of an efficient

oar should be beyond Point A but not too far. See Oar Efficiency (section 14).

Bear in mind with these slip diagrams that the boat's forward motion is only accomplished by the reaction of the mass of water propelled directly aft by the blade. Who knows whether Sir Isaac Newton ever rowed a boat, but he was the first to perceive this reaction mathematically. Water moved laterally by the blade (with respect to the boat's forward motion) only reacts thwartwise on the locks to bend the gunwales and represents wasted energy. For maximum oar efficiency, the lateral blade thrust on the locks should be kept at a minimum as will be explained later. The one time during a stroke when there is the least lateral movement of water by a flat blade, is when the oar is thwartwise. But we cannot row with the oar always held there so the overall propulsion efficiency of the entire stroke must be less than the momentary efficiency while the oar is thwartwise. And short strokes, with their lessened lateral movement of water in the puddles by the blade, are more efficient than long strokes. All of this reasoning can be read in slip diagrams.

The slip diagrams yield the further information that a double pair-oared boat can use harder pulling oars, because it is moving faster, than when driven by a single pair. The second rower presumably doubles the available power. However, depending on the boat, the extra displacement will absorb most of the added power so perhaps the boat will go only 10% to 20% faster. Thus the distance r, from lock to Point A in the expression r=12V/m could be made 10% to 20% longer. So assuming 8′-long single pair oars to start with, the outer looms of the double pairs can be made about 5" to 9" longer for the same boat.

A cautionary note: Since the slip diagrams apply only to

boat speed through the water and not to speed over the bottom, river and tidal currents are irrelevant to slip.

While slip is desirable in lessening the shock load on the rower's body, it is also the chief culprit responsible for propulsion losses. But then, if we didn't have a fluid medium for oars to slip in, we wouldn't have boats either. The energy losses in the oar puddles, which can be reduced with good oar design, will be considered in future sections.

{7}

Oar Fit in the Locks

A free but close and silent fit of the oars in the locks is a real pleasure, eases the shock load of the pull on the rower, gives better control of the blades, provides closer harmony with the water, and reduces lock wear. Any effort to correct excessive looseness is warranted for all but casual rowing. Metal to metal swivel locks should be kept greased always or the shanks and sockets will grow egg shaped and get progressively worse. For feathering oars the leathers should be a close running fit between the yoke horns and be lubricated if the material requires it. A close fit also reduces wear on the buttons if present. Of course locks such as the double thole cannot be tightened.

Polished brass (bronze for salt water) single-thole-pin locks of the St. Lawrence skiff with a leathered slot-hole in the oar are the quietest, cleanest, and easiest to maintain. The Adirondack guide boat lock is the next easiest to maintain if the shank is greased each time the boat is taken for a row. It has no leather. However, these two lock types won't feather so they are preferred only by the local connoisseurs and scorned by the multitudes elsewhere. The feathering swivel yoke lock is the hardest to maintain. The amount of lock sloppiness can't be easily measured and stated in numbers, but there is no doubt that a good boat and oars with sloppy locks will come to life when the locks are corrected.

{8}
Overlap of Grips

This requires cross handed rowing, preferred by some folks and disdained by others. I was raised without incident on cornmeal mush and overlap. Not until later, in other parts of the country, was scorn heaped upon both matters.

Overlap may occur when oars having long enough inner looms to properly propel the boat happen to be put in comparatively narrow inland, or other craft under 46" to 48" beam, such as the Adirondack, St. Lawrence, and small Rangeley boats. With few exceptions, these traditional boats do not have folding or outrigger locks, which would increase lock span and could avoid overlap. Shortening the inner looms to avoid overlap makes oars harder to pull and balance. Once inner loom length is determined for propulsion reasons it should be but slightly compromised, if at all. Why some boats are beamier than others is naturally outside the scope of this article.

Although at times there seems to be a conflict here between oars and boat beam that is resolved by overlap, there is a real physical benefit to be had with some overlap. The reasons are that the rower's hands are not so far apart at either end of the stroke so he has better control of the oars and, on the average, his body lines up better with the grips. Sometimes a strong pull on one oar is needed to correct a boat's course and it is easier for the rower to pull hard if he can get his skeleton in line with the grip. Due to the sideways arc the grip travels, the rower must compromise anyway to line himself up. But with some overlap, the grips will line up better for most of the stroke.

The coastal rower, conditioned to beamier boats without

overlap, is usually uncomfortable in the inland boats, but his hands can coordinate and adapt to overlap if his brain will let them. Admittedly, the lack of feathering in many inland boats makes cross-handed rowing easier. Overlaps of 4" to 8" are often seen and can be managed. The most non-feathering overlap I've measured and seen in action is 15" in a 36" beam Adirondack guide boat. See oar #13 in Table 1. The keen rower was rangy, had long arms, and sprouted from a guide boat at an early age.

The limit to overlap is an individual matter determined by how long the rower's arms and torso are, his midships girth, and the bulkiness of his clothes. It is determined when the ends of the oars dig him in the ribs or foul his clothes. Too much overlap for a particular person forces him to sit too far forward of the locks and hunker over the oars. It also tends to shorten his stroke because he wants to get the oars out of the water before they get him in the ribs! If he sits too far forward his stroke becomes too unsymmetrical, with not enough of it at the beginning and too much at the end. A dandy illustration of successful non-feathering high overlap (probably 12") is shown in WoodenBoat #18, page 57 - a guide boat in racing trim. The oars are #13 in Table 1. There are no clothes to snag the oars. Also note how limber these soft maple oars are. While a guide-boat wake is flat at cruising speed, this boat is shown with considerable wave action, indicating that she is stepping right along.

I don't know of any simple formula to determine maximum overlap. Each rower has to try what he can tolerate. Locks that fold outward in service, although requiring care, can be a solution for some relatively narrow boats in reducing but not eliminating overlap if there is sea room to swing the oars and the extra lock weight is tolerable for portaging.

The gist of overlap is not to let it interfere with oar design. Treat overlap, if any, as a problem in the rower's coordination, build, and temperament and move the locks outward as the boat and conditions allow. Just remember to keep your thumbs off the oar ends, and with high overlap keep your knuckles away from the opposite loom, particularly if the loom is enlarged and the boat is lively on rough water. All of this comes naturally to those well versed in the art. Greater overlap, especially in tender boats, slows maximum stroke rate unless the oarsman is very experienced. I have timed 56 spm for about 12" overlap, non-feathering of course, during a guide-boat race.

The foregoing concerns straight blades. But it is seen later in <u>Oar Efficiency</u> (section 14) that the tip angle of a spoon blade forces the whole arc of blade travel toward the bow and the rower toward the stern. Consequently less overlap may be desirable with spoon oars than with straight blades in a fixed-seat boat. A sliding seat allows more overlap with spoons as the rower's midriff moves away from the oars during the pull. I can manage 4-1/4" overlap with spoon oars #43 with a fixed seat. Being a grandfather, maybe a small rocking chair would allow me more overlap.

{9}

Handle Shapes

Handle sizes and shapes show such inconceivable variety the world around that obviously there is no best way. Local tradition seems most influential, and the adaptability of the human hand allows the survival of weird shapes, after the callouses are developed. But a sticky surface should be avoided, and a cylindrical grip, or nearly so, is easy to make.

To fashion an oar quickly and easily by hand, long cutting strokes are needed. With the feathering oar enlarged for strength at the lock, this sometimes leads to a round tapered inner loom with the grip an extension of it. So the grip may be slightly conical instead of cylindrical. However, the non-feathering oar is generally square or rectangular at the lock, and this shape often persists along the inner loom for extra weight to help counterweight the oar. The shape of the grip is then not influenced by the shaping of the inner loom. The feathering oar with square inner counterbalance loom seems to be a hybrid and is more trouble to make because of the change to a round section at both the lock and grip.

It would seem sensible that the size of the rower's hand should determine the grip diameter, although this is mostly not the case. A cylindrical grip 1-9/16" to 1-3/4" diameter by 5" long fits me fine. This is a larger diameter than many prefer, but it distributes the pull over greater skin area with less tendency to blister. The larger diameter also allows excavation for balancing lead in the grip, and up to a point gives the hand better leverage when rolling a feathering oar. If it is too big, it can be worked down. Guide-boat grips are made very small and conical (large end at end of oar). One stated reason being that there is then

less knuckle interference with the opposing loom of these high overlap oars in these very tiddly boats. A lot of gloves are worn these days in guide boats to prevent blisters and bruises. But the Adirondack folks swear by their small grips.

For a long row, some folks prefer non-feathering locks as there is no lost rolling wrist energy and a loose grip is possible on both the pull and recovery strokes. In fact, with a balanced oar in a non-feathering lock, the fingers can be momentarily flexed on the recovery and the hand can roam around on the grip. Such an oar can be rowed with thumb and pinky when things are right. In contrast, a feathering oar must be continuously grasped.

Most rowers prefer the lower windage advantage of feathering. But many automatically feather in a calm, and in going down wind. This is a sad sight indeed, a pleasure rower whose reflexes have been too well conditioned, when he could leave the oar unfeathered and "sail" it down a strong wind.

{10}

Stroke Length and Rate

As the angle of a straight bladed oar departs from its thwartwise position, the effectiveness of the blade in moving water aft diminishes and the oar becomes less efficient at moving the boat forward. The effectiveness varies as the cosine of the angle of departure from thwartwise, and is shown by the cosine curve in figure 2. Thus, a given amount of human energy applied when the oar is thwartwise is more effective than when applied at the stroke ends. If the rower has energy to burn, he can lengthen his stroke and thereby get more energy into it. But if he uses the same amount of extra energy either when the oar is thwartwise, or to quicken his short stroke, he will travel farther. Like other aspects of rowing there is no simple number to put on how long a stroke should be. This is something each rower must determine for himself by trial and error.

Short fast strokes with an easy pulling oar show up best when going to windward. A rower should be in good condition though to tackle a strong headwind with that stroke, and should pace himself for the distance according to his stamina, because this is like racing.

It is fascinating to examine photographs and movies of rowers in action. Sometimes one sees the start or end of a long pull when it is very evident that the oar is not at an efficient angle. Sometimes a straight bladed oar is seen at an angle of 45 degrees or more from thwartwise when its position efficiency is only 71% or less.

Another aspect of the long stroke is that more back motion is needed and thus more transfer of the rower's weight fore and aft, and a greater tendency to bob the boat's bow up

and down. If an extra yank is pulled at the end of the stroke, the bow is driven even deeper. Light and short boats with fine waterlines, such as some guide boats, are the most susceptible bobbers of the fixed seat boats and particularly so when rowed from the forward seat (thwart to coastal folk). Nobody appears to know exactly how much extra hull resistance the bobbing action produces, but the surges readily seen in the bow wave don't look like energy savers. For easy rowing and to husband energy, a fairly short stroke with maximum pull in the middle, and little body motion seems to produce a more uniform boat motion, but it requires more arm action and better arm condition.

For a day's row there is no one best stroke rate because the condition of the wind, water, and rower will change. So it behooves the rower to adapt to a wide range in stroke rate and style. Naturally some of us older folks will start off easy and sometimes end that way too. I have loafed for several hours with an easy-running boat at moderate speed at 15 short easy strokes per minute with basically hard-pulling oars (#31B in Table 1), starting in a daybreak calm. In this mode the boat eats up very little energy and the miles slide by. Where we are now soon becomes way back yonder in the blue. Then later it might be necessary to go up to 50 short spm with the easy-pulling oars (#43B) to get around some point of land against the wind and a strong river current. Rowing as low as 15 spm has a peculiar feel at first and requires some steady practice to adapt to it. Once achieved, it comes naturally if the pull is not too hard. It is a hurry-up-and-wait stroke with a relatively fast, short pull and a slower recovery.

I have not seen any test data on the resistance and power needed to move a rowboat with a cyclic velocity due to periodic stroking. Since the water mass carried along in the boundary layer by the boat's skin friction is affected,

as well as the pulsing of energy put into the wave systems, I would guess that non-uniform boat velocity would increase the boat's total resistance and that the increase percentage-wise would be greater with slower strokes, which would produce a greater range of variation in boat speed. I can't prove this thesis with numbers, but if it is so, it favors shorter and faster strokes. However, at low loafing speeds, where there isn't much energy at stake and total boat resistance is relatively low, the hurry up and wait stroke seems to work. But this stroke won't work against a strong wind. Then the recovery should be as fast as possible to get the oar back in the water to retain the boat's speed, still using a short stroke as the most efficient. Naturally this leads to a fast stroke with basically easy-pulling oars. Using short strokes for either easy or hard going means that the stroke rate is greatly affected by the relative length of time of the recovery. This variable style requires practice to get used to. At intermediate stroke rates the length of time for the pull and recovery will be more nearly equal, so a more uniform stroke rhythm results. This will be the case over a wide range of boat speeds except the extreme conditions mentioned.

A deliberate change of gait is refreshing. One way is to "dog paddle" for a spell. While this slows the boat speed a little, it works well in an easy-running boat. The alternate side stroking is short and at a higher rate, and there is less transfer of rower's weight fore and aft. Consequently, the boat moves smoothly with less surging and bobbing, all of which seems to be a more efficient way of using the rower's energy. This stroke seems to work better with non-feathering oars.

Occasionally, even the non-racing rower finds either by choice or necessity that he must move the oars with the

utmost alacrity. If the oars are feathering, they should roll in their locks with the greatest of ease, lest too much of the rower's energy be dissipated in rolling his wrists and in a tight grip. In this respect the non-feathering lock allows an advantage of sustaining a higher stroke rate than a feathered oar. The racing fellows in the Adirondacks, where locks are non-feathering, say they lack time to feather at 55 spm, and ensure that on every grab the blade enters the water at exactly the best angle. Also, the high overlap of these oars would make them harder to feather.

A tuned oar of the lightest weight consistent with adequate strength, and hence with minimum counterweight, if any, and the least required inertia force, can be moved faster than a heavy oar. So it needs less energy to move at a given rate, whether the lock feathers or not, and in a tight situation a tuned oar may be a safer oar to get the rower quickly out of harm's way.

Movies of rowers are a lively source of information on how oars and boats are used. Those who like racing have a dandy chance to see how the other fellow does it, observing things that might not be noticed during the excitement of the race. Movies of a succession of annual rowing races are of interest to local winter gatherings. A variable-speed projector helps.

(Note: The above section was written over 10 years ago. A new complementary section (25) Synchronizing the Rower's To-and-Fro Motion appears later in this tale to benefit vigorous rowers who must put more "back" into a stronger stroke.)

{11}

Leverage

This is another fun subject because there are at least four leverage systems involved in rowing. The reader sometimes must figure out from the context what system a writer is dealing with. First, there is the geometric ratio of the length of oar outboard of the lock to the length inboard. This ratio lacks functional meaning. Second is the motion lever of that part of the oar momentarily connecting the lock to the "water pivot" Point A, seen only when the oar is thwartwise, and previously described under Slip (section 6). Third is a force lever shown in figure 3, which is the ratio of the distance between lock and blade center of pressure, q, to the distance between lock and grip center, (B-2"). Fourth is a turning lever that the rower uses with his oars to change course. This will be dealt with later.

For the force lever, the center of water pressure on the blade is difficult to locate exactly because the dynamic water pressure is not uniformly distributed over the entire blade due to varying local slip velocities and blade shape. Since the tip region is the most effective, the c.p. will lie somewhere between the tip and the geometric center of the blade. We will assume the c.p. lies 1/5 of the blade length inward from the tip. The total equivalent water force applied perpendicularly to the blade and taken at its c.p. times the force lever ratio, and plus lock friction, will be the force of the water transmitted to the rower's hand. I am unaware of any data of this nature for pleasure oars but it would be useful for classifying hard- and easy-pulling oars.

I have tinkered with a crude expression to rate the pulling intensity of an oar: Y=RxW; where R is a simplified force lever defined as a ratio: (distance between lock and tip

minus an arbitrary 1/5 blade length) to (B-2"); and W is maximum blade width in inches. See figure 3. It is assumed that the blade force is roughly proportional to maximum blade width at some constant comparative slip for all oars. Obviously, the resulting dimensions of Y are inches and not pounds as they should be. So in this case the pull number, Y, is given its appropriate designation for an unknown quantity, in keeping with its mongrel status. I hope some reader can do better on a simple basis. Y is shown in column 21 for the oars listed in Table 1. Perhaps the usefulness of Y might be in designing a new oar with a different pull than the one which a rower is presently familiar with for a certain boat. However, the idea is experimental and should be used with judgement. It probably works best on similarly shaped blades. (More on this later.)

Force lever ratio, R, is shown for ready reference among the formulae on Table 1, and for comparison in column 20. By itself, this ratio doesn't mean much, except that a very high value, such as R=4.0 for oar #24, may show a hard pulling oar. The main usefulness of R is in conjunction with blade width W, to estimate the pull number Y.

{12}
Inner Loom Length

Functionally, this is the distance (B-2"), figure 3, and it affects oar characteristics in many ways. From a detached viewpoint a rower simply has a short lever in his grasp extending only to the lock and which is worked to and fro in a particular path. For a given action at the blade the princples of leverage say the pull intensity at the grip is inversely proportional to inner loom length. For an extreme example, a very short inner loom, say half the length the rower is accustomed to, will make him pull twice as hard through half the distance, and his skeleton and the skin on his hands might complain. Note that since the blade action is assumed the same, the work done by the blade on the water (work equals force times distance the force moves) is the same regardless of inner loom length. However, the rower's efficiency is highest at some particular inner loom length that best suits his physique.

Tall rowers with long arms can have more fore-and-aft reach of their hands than short rowers with short arms. So the longer-armed rower should have oars with longer inner looms in order to keep the angle of swing of the oars from being excessive which would result in lower efficiency (see figure 2). This also suggests that long-armed rowers should have wider lock spans to keep the grip overlap from being excessive (see Overlap of Grips, section 8). If a short-armed rower gets into a boat with oars designed for a tall rower, he can still manage to the limit of his comfortable fore-and-aft reach. The swing angle of the oars will be less and hence more efficient for the whole stroke. However, if a long-armed rower gets into a short man's boat, he will find that he cannot reach fore and aft to his own limit without getting into excessive swing angle and losing some efficiency. He will be cramped.

Note also that this idea of matching the inner loom length to the rower's reach is seen in sliding-seat boats, which have oars with inner looms about 33" to 34" long to utilize the longer reach afforded by the slide. For the same pull intensity and angle of swing, these longer inner looms allow more work to be gotten from longer outer looms and wider blades.

So the question is what is the best inner loom length for a particular rower in a fixed-seat boat. There is no simple answer. Each rower will have to figure it out for himself. But he should try to keep the inner loom as long as he can manage. Maybe column 4 in Table 1 will help. My regular oars are #43 & #31 with B=25-1/2". Oars #1 are ladies' oars, which small children have learned to row with. My experience (I'm 6' tall) is that B shouldn't be less than 25" to 26", and I believe I could readily manage a few more inches if the lock span is also increased. The outer part of an oar cannot be designed to do a lot of work with a normal pull intensity if the inner loom is too short.

The idea of having maximum length inner looms applies not only to oars with larger outboard dimensions suitable for downwind rowing but also to upwind oars with smaller outboard dimensions. In fact, it is for the tougher rowing upwind that long inner looms are most necessary. By this concept, if one has several different pairs of oars for his own use, they should all be about the same maximum inner loom length regardless of the outboard dimensions. One encounters the old rule in various forms, that an oar should have a certain ratio of outboard to inboard lengths. Such rules don't withstand analytical scrutiny. The design of oars is covered in greater detail in a later installment.

Reverting to the discussion of Leverage (section 11), and the simplified expression for pull number, Y=RxW, a simplified work number, WN, of an oar can be obtained, if Y is multiplied by the distance the grip moves. Since that distance is proportional to the inner loom length (B-2") for a given angle of swing, we can simplify the work number further and say WN=Yx(B-2")=RxWx(B-2"). Since R=(A-B-BL/5)/(B-2") then mathematically, WN=(A-B-BL/5)xW, which says in another way that unless the outer loom is lengthened and/or the blade widened, we cannot get more work out of an oar for a given slip and angle of swing just by making the inner loom longer. Table 1, column 22, shows the work number of some oars.

The commercial spruce feathering spoon oar #24A in Table 1 is an interesting example of too short an inner loom. This oar could be improved by using the knowledge in this article and would then become a pleasure to use and an asset to the boat. The length of the oar is 7′, and the inner loom is 17-1/2" if rowed on the button. The pull number is very high at Y=21.4, but its work number is only moderately low at WN=334. So, this oar is very hard to pull but doesn't do commensurate work. Also, it is far out of balance with P=4.4 lbs., and it is very stiff. The trouble seems to be that the inner loom length of this oar has been pinched to fit a narrow boat without overlap. If the inner loom was spliced out to 22-1/2" (still a bit short) without changing the button location, the pull number would drop to a respectable 16.2, which equals 21.4x(17.5-2)/(22.5-2), and the unbalanced P would drop to 3.3 lbs. which would still require thinning the blade and outer loom and possible some counterweighting. The overlap would change from nothing to about 7" when the oars are used in the 14′-7" Rangeley shown. If this overlap seems excessive to some folks, then move the locks outward.

Incidentally, this boat is one of my favorite small, one-man double-enders. It goes beautifully for a short boat. The movies of it in action show very little fuss on the water when it is moving smartly. It has a good workable compromise between initial lateral stability and speed. Its wetted surface is fairly low, being 27 sq. ft. with one rower (165 lbs. for rower plus 125 lbs. for boat and oars). It was originally built by Ellis and has been replicated many times over by Mystic Seaport Museum's Small Boat Shop. For those interested, complete construction drawings are available reasonably through the Museum's Ships' Plans Division, Box 6000, Mystic, CT 06355-0990. I think this little wooden rowboat is one of the gems of our nautical heritage for pleasure rowing.

To summarize, a longer inner loom will do the following and a shorter one the opposite, all assuming the rest of the oar is unchanged:

1. Balance an oar easier with the weight of rower's hand;

2. Decrease the inertia force, F, at the grip due to oar inertia and acceleration;

3. Reduce the pull intensity on the grip due to a given blade action in the water;

4. Increase the to-and-fro travel of the grip for a given angle of swing;

5. Increase the grip overlap for a given lock spread, or require an increase in lock spread for a given overlap;

6. Make rowing easier and consume less rower's energy

if the inner loom is too short to begin with and the pull too hard;

7. Require more rower's energy if the inner loom is already too long and the pull too easy;

8. Allow more work to be put into a stroke if the outer loom length and/or blade width is increased and the rower can stand it. This will result in higher boat speed, a stronger turning lever, and better boat maneuverability.

Going back to the turning lever, it exists when the rower pulls harder on one oar than the other to alter course. A double turn stroke backs one oar and pulls on the other. The turning motion of a boat already underway is complicated, but it is obvious that one stroke of a high-work-number oar will turn the boat farther than a low-work-number oar.

{13}

Boat Maneuverability

Good maneuverability depends on good boat design as well as on high-work-number oars. Of course, a boat can be turned with more strokes of lower-work-number oars, but sometimes these strokes must be made in a big hurry. Often a rowboat is least maneuverable when going to leeward in quartering wind and waves, and particularly when surfing when it is most likely to broach. This is the time when high-work-number oars will get the boat back on course and put zip into a responsive boat.

A rough test in still water of the combined maneuverability of boat and oars is to begin with a standing start and count the number of full double-turning strokes to spin the boat 360 degrees. There is quite a variation among different boats and oars. If a boat can be turned completely around once in 6 double strokes, it is very maneuverable. If it takes a dozen or more strokes, it is sluggish.

Maneuverability in broken water requires far different rowing technique than the highly perfected uniform stroking used by racing shell oarsmen in smooth water. In rough water, hardly any two successive strokes are alike. It is catch as catch can with many ragged strokes, late catches, a few clean misses, many short strokes, and uneven pulls to straighten the course. Sometimes a rower must synchronize with the waves when they grow as big as the boat, all while the boat is moving in all its degrees of freedom of motion. Light, balanced, and limber oars that can be quickly and surely moved are good shipmates. Plenty of experience is the best teacher, and the more experience, the more fun. Double-oared rowing in rough water upwind is very effective in moving the boat fast enough to pound at times.

{14}

Oar Efficiency

Let's dive head first into this subject, hoping that by now the water is neither too cold for the reader nor too hot for the writer. Figure 4 shows an oar at some arbitrary instant with the forces on it at grip, lock, and J, lbs. at the blade center of pressure. The oar is turning with an angular velocity, m, radians/sec. The distance from lock to c.p. is q inches, and the angle of the oar to thwartwise is h deg. The tangential velocity of the c.p. is U, ft./sec.=mxq/12. The boat is moving ahead with velocity, V, ft./sec. The useful component of J in the direction the boat moves is Jxcos(h). Let power at that instant equal force times velocity, ft.-lbs./sec. The total oar efficiency, (TE), is power absorbed by boat's forward motion which is VxJxcos(h), divided by power input into the oar. With JxU the power into the blade and (LE) the oarlock efficiency, the power into the oar is JxU/(LE). Combining, (TE)=(LE)x(V/U)xcos(h). Call V/U a velocity efficiency =(VE), and cos(h) a position efficiency =(PE). Then (TE)=(LE)x(VE)x(PE). So, to get the total oar propulsive efficiency, all we have to do is multiply the three different efficiency components together. We can also examine each component separately in order to get a better idea of how improvements can be made.

The lock efficiency, (LE), is high with a well lubricated lock. The efficiency of the non-feathering lock such as the single thole pin of the St. Lawrence skiff and the pinned yoke of the guide boat is the highest, maybe 97%, and there is not much potential improvement. A feathering lock by itself can be as mechanically efficient as the two above locks. However, the feathering lock demands additional energy from the rower that is not needed by the others because the rower must roll his wrists and keep a tighter

grasp throughout the whole stroke. The non-feathering lock permits a relaxed grip on the return stroke, and the rower needn't be concerned about the proper blade angle at every catch. A feathering oar such as the racers use, with a flat side bearing against a straight horn at the correct blade angle, and which has a natural or synthetic "leather" as slippery as an eel, is a decided improvement for pleasure rowing. But even then it requires more energy than the non-feathering oar. But the non-feathering lock offsets its disadvantages by making it easier to reach the higher stroke rates with a more dependable precision on the catch, which then results in better utilization of the rower's major effort. Each rower has his "druthers," usually stated emphatically and invariably dependent on where he was raised and on his favorite type of lock. I don't know anybody who has forsaken the non-feathering lock for a feathering one, but several friends have converted to non-feathering locks because they are easier to use and need less energy.

Position efficiency, (PE), depends on how far the oar is from thwartwise. This was mentioned under <u>Stroke Length and Rate</u> (section 10), see figure 2. Here the rower has some control over oar efficiency depending on the stroke length he chooses. (PE) is 100% when a straight bladed oar is thwartwise, and diminishes as the stroke angle each side of thwartwise increases.

Now, the interesting one is velocity efficiency, (VE), which is the ratio of boat velocity to the tangential velocity of the blade c.p. with respect to the lock. V/U will always be less than 1.0 for normal pulls, and note that it depends on the combination of boat speed, oar, and rower. Once the boat, oar, wind, and water conditions are set, the rower's control to maintain high (VE) depends on his skill to keep as much way on as possible, particularly

in adverse conditions. If he lets the boat stop so V is zero, then (VE) and the total oar efficiency, (TE), also are zero. This is the case if the boat's stern painter is still tied to the dock, see figure 1a, or when starting underway at the beginning of the first pull, or when a blast of headwind stops the boat. The rower is diligently putting the power in, but the boat, "she-no-go." This is also the time when the slip velocity is greatest. If V equaled U, then (VE) would be 1.0 (or 100%), but this cannot happen because then there would be no slip and so no blade pressure. Another way to regard (VE) is that it depends on slip, and the less the slip, the greater the velocity efficiency, (VE), becomes. If we look at the oar when thwartwise and (PE) is 1.0, it is also noted that V/U is the same as the ratio of r/q=(VE), see figure 4. So as r moves in and out along the loom with the water pivot Point A, depending on conditions related previously, so does (VE) vary. We would like r as far out and/or q as far in as possible while we have an acceptable stroke rate. When the boat is running easily, r does move outward (see slip figure 1d), and the total propulsive efficiency of the oar, (TE), increases. When the boat is running adversely, the opposite occurs. One good way to get higher propulsive efficiency is to look for a faster boat. Among the traditional fixed-seat craft, the Adirondack guide boat allows the highest potential oar propulsive efficiency because its higher inherent boat speed moves the water pivot Point A outward, thus increasing r/q and the velocity efficiency. As far as velocity efficiency is concerned, the guide boat acts like a slower boat with a strong wind behind it (see slip figure 1d again). In both cases Point A moves closer to the blade c.p. An extreme example is the single racing shell which runs so fast that pt. A has moved out so far that oars with much longer outer loom dimension from lock to blade neck are needed, the distance being in the neighborhood of 64". The oars for these craft have very

good velocity efficiencies because the c.p. is relatively so close to Point A.

Combining the oar efficiency with the rower's efficiency, (RE), the overall efficiency (soup to knots) is (OE)=(RE)x(LE)x(PE)x(VE), and it is noted that (RE), (PE), and (VE) all vary during the stroke so that (OE) will probably vary also. What is needed is the best overall combination of efficiencies for the total stroke. I don't know exactly how the rower's efficiency varies during the stroke, but presumably it is least at the ends when he is changing direction and best when the oar is near thwartwise where (PE) is also highest. Since the pulsing motion of the oars produces some surging in the boat's velocity, the velocity efficiency probably also varies, being higher in the latter part of the stroke than earlier when the boat is slower. So it seems that taking the three major efficiencies, (RE), (PE), and (VE), in combination, the most efficient part of the stroke for a straight blade is probably just as the oar passes thwartwise. If so, this is the best time to pull harder, rather than during other parts of the stroke.

The above reasoning applies only to straight-bladed oars in fixed seat boats. If the oar is a spoon, then the whole pulling stroke arc at the blade should be moved forward by an amount in degrees equal to the angle the tip makes with respect to the long oar axis (see figure 5). Then the most efficient part of the stroke is in the fore stroke, demonstrating that spoon oars should be rowed differently than straight-bladed oars.

The idea that the dynamic velocity efficiency, (VE), when the oar is thwartwise, equals r/q with the oars and boat in motion, can be extended to a similar idea of static oar proportions when the water pivot Point A is at the blade

neck. This will occur under certain conditions of boat speed and angular oar velocity. If we arbitrarily set r equal to the distance from lock to neck, and since q already equals the distance from lock to blade center of pressure, then we can define a Base Oar Efficiency, (BE)=(A-B-BL)/(A-B-BL/5). It will be recalled from Table 1, that A is overall oar length, B is distance from lock to grip end, and BL is blade length. Here, as previously assumed, the blade c.p. is at a distance BL/5 inward from the tip. Thus, (BE) characterizes the oar's dimensions and allows comparison with other oars, even though they are not in motion. Since the velocity efficiency, (VE)=r/q, increases or decreases as the water pivot Point A moves outward or inward respectively, according to motion conditions, then (VE) will only equal (BE) when the water pivot is at the neck. Column 23 in Table 1 lists (BE) for the various oars. The reader can easily figure (BE) for his own oars and compare with his friends and the table.

Figure 6 shows graphically the relation of (BE) to the outer oar length dimensions. It is seen that greater base oar efficiency occurs with longer outer oar length and shorter (but wider) blades because the neck is relatively closer to the blade c.p. This also means that longer outer oars and/or wider blades will have a higher work number, WN, which sparks another idea that (BE) might be a function of WN. Very neatly this turns out to be so in figure 7. This derivation is not given here, but it can be done by those interested with the equations shown on Table 1, where it is arbitrarily defined that Q=WxBL. Figure 7 shows that for constant Q, higher-work-number oars have higher base oar efficiency. Q is the convenient but fictitious "block area" of a rectangle of width W enclosing the blade. Later, under Selection of Oars (section 16), a family of 4 standardized blades of different widths and lengths will be used in an example. All 4 blades happen to have about the

same Q.

The idea of base oar efficiency can be applied to the suggestion that two different pairs of oars be carried on a long row - one pair with a lower pull number, work number, and base oar efficiency, and the other pair with higher values of these three characteristics. It is then evident that when the boat wants to run easily, say downwind, switching to the higher-number oars will have the added benefit of possibly reaching higher propulsive efficiency and further conserving the rower's energy.

Of course, we should have as efficient oars as possible, whether they have low or high pull and work numbers. But as figure 6 shows, oars with shorter outer looms that are more suited for upwind rowing will have lower base efficiency compared to oars with longer outboard looms and usually higher pull and work numbers, all oars so compared to have the same blade length on the graph.

{15}
Blade Area and Shape

What sort of pleasure oar blade shall we pick for our use from the vast assortment humans have created? I haven't found any published test data on the effectiveness of long narrow vs. short wide blades; spoon vs. flat blades; or the best shape and curvature of spoons. Subjective opinion, however, flourishes indeed. The slow trial and error racing approach led to the modern, short wide racing spoon blade as the most efficient shape yet devised. But the question is whether the spoon is worth the extra cost and work to build over a flat blade for pleasure rowing. To some folks the spoon's shape is aesthetically pleasing. Others who like to row a lot prefer the spoon's higher efficiency.

A good spoon oar has better attention paid to blade shape, balance, length, and selection of light material than the ordinary flat-bladed oar. Yet, if equal pains are taken to make and tune a flat-bladed pleasure oar with blade outline similar to the spoon but with another 1/4" to 1/2" width, if possible, and a shorter blade, it will work nearly as well and will be easier to make than the spoon. Full-feathering spoon blades are required to stabilize narrow racing shells, but that isn't needed for our purposes.

The spoon blade has a higher propulsion efficiency due to its curvature, so it is a better converter of the rower's energy into forward boat motion. My guess is that slip figure 1g provides a clue. Since the slip velocity of the water coming into the blade endwise on the fore stroke is at an oblique angle, some blade curvature at the tip will let the water enter with less eddy loss and move the center of water pressure (the sweet spot) closer to the water pivot Point A, which must happen if the propulsion

efficiency is higher than for a straight blade. Higher efficiency is a fine recommendation for a spoon for distance rowing.

We can reason why the modern, short wide blade has higher propulsion efficiency than the older, long narrow blade, even disregarding the spoon curvature and considering both as flat blades. Reverting to Oar Efficiency (section 14), the velocity efficiency component of propulsion efficiency provides the key, since (VE)=r/q. This means that the blade center of pressure should be inboard, as close to the water pivot Point A as possible, i.e., a short but necessarily wide blade. See figures 1c and 4, also.

The limit to a wider blade is the ease of getting the blade cleanly in and out of the water and over the wave tops. Up to 6" and 7" blade width can be handled with racing spoons in rough open-water races. Structurally, the wider blades have been made for over a half century without an expensive wide board, simply by laminating together a wide blade assembly.

The sprint racer wants to get there "fustest," the pleasure and long-distance rowers the easiest, and the long distance racer, the "fustest" and the easiest. They all talk the same high efficiency language because the "engine" is so weak.

Efficient spoon oars are not restricted to fast boats. They can be used at all boat speeds with a suitable length outer loom and stroke rate. We have seen that the distance, r, from lock to water pivot Point A equals 12V/m. Then r is proportional to boat speed, V, and inversely proportional to instantaneous stroke rate, m, which is mostly a characteristic of the rower's style. So at normal stroke rates we can have short, wide, efficient spoon or flat

blades on short outer looms for slow boats, and on longer looms for faster boats. Also, highly efficient racing spoon oars with wide short blades on long outer looms have been used at slow stroke rates to cross oceans at slow boat speeds.

Since high propulsion efficiency is associated with low slip and consequently greater blade area, it is easy to spot a high efficiency oar by its generous blade area lumped at the end of the loom rather than stretched out in a long blade. A very small blade, though, has a suspicious look. It will have a high slip and low efficiency for an adult pull.

Non-feathering oars will enter the water at a consistent angle. If this angle is set to "dig" about 2 degrees (see figure 8) when fitting the oar to the lock, the oar won't jump the lock on a hard pull, and the rower never has to fiddle with the proper blade angle. However, this particular angle doesn't apply to oars for racing shells where the situation is different. Non-feathering oars set to "dig" with the blade axis at an angle to the vertical become permanently right and left handed, as a little reflection will reveal.

During the fore stroke, when the blade tip is moving outward into the water (see slip figure 1g), a wider tip can take better advantage of this scooping motion than a narrower one, and particularly if it is a curved spoon blade. The tip edge, it seems, should be thin and straight with the corners only slightly rounded to better withstand wear and tear.

One sometimes sees a very-long-bladed spoon oar, often much narrower at the tip than in its mid portion. It is hard to see how there can be much scooping in the fore stroke with

such a narrow tip. While the oar may look handsome to some folks, the labor in making the spoon shape could probably have been better spent in tuning a flat oar by lightening the blade and outer loom and adding counterweights if necessary.

Note that blade area doesn't enter directly into the pull and work numbers as shown by comparing columns 13, 21, and 22 in Table 1. A review of other oar data in addition to Table 1 shows that blade areas between 105 and 120 sq. in. are adequate for short wide blades, whether spoon or flat, with blade lengths between 19" and 26" and widths 5-1/2" to 7-1/2", with the wider blades matching the shorter.

Mr. Douglas Martin has mentioned the hydrodynamic aspect of the doryman's short, choppy stroke with considerable dipping down and up through the water. During descent and ascent the blade acts like an aerofoil giving an added forward thrust (see figure 9). The center of water pressure on the blade for this action is closer to the water pivot Point A than the c.p. due to the fore-and-aft sweeping action, so there is an increased propulsion efficiency with the doryman's stroke. Also, there is a little firmer bite with less fore-and-aft slip, and consequently lower puddle losses. This action also moves Point A slightly outward with another small increase of boat speed. The blade cross-section should be an efficient, smooth, reversible aerofoil, rather flat or slightly concave on the after or pressure face and crowned on the bow or suction face. Obviously, the long, narrow blades having a handsome ridge down the middle of one or both faces are not as efficient as dipping aerofoils, and the ridges splash on entering and leaving the water. The deep dipping requires more vertical hand motion and some vertically expended work. Also, there is some energy loss of the loom backing water on the deeper dips.

The doryman's stroke is good at low power, but at higher power more fore-and-aft energy is needed, and the short wide blade is better. A composite stroke is very desirable using various proportions of dipping with the horizontal sweeping motion, and such a stroke adds to the rower's repertoire of strokes to play on his oars.

To sum up blade shape, the rower's spent energy is displayed before him and can be seen, heard, and felt. In today's idiom, "It all hangs out." He can see his energy lost in the puddles, in the boat's bow, quarter, and transverse stern waves, and in the boundary layer turbulence in the wake. He may hear the bow wave and oar splashing. He feels air resistance on himself, the oars, and the boat. And he feels and hears the boat bucking into head waves. The kinetic energy loss in the oar puddles depends on the amount of water disturbed in them and the square of the velocity imparted to it by the blades. The gist of the best shape and manner of use of the blades is to transfer as much energy loss as possible from the puddles over to the boat's loss system. The puddle loss can be reduced by disturbing a larger quantity of water with the blade but at a lower velocity. Thus, minimum slip is desired and is accomplished with short blades having enough area, which means wide blades. Stronger rowers need more blade area and width in order to reduce slip and puddle loss.

Also, submerge the blades far enough so water doesn't visibly wash over their tops with cavitation (an air pocket behind the blade, which gives a softer, "washed out" pull and more slip). Dig deeper with the stronger pulls. The doryman's added submergence into deeper water at greater pressure prevents cavitation and allows the blade to disturb even more water with consequently lower water

velocity and less puddle loss. A large, active surface disturbance in the puddle is a sign of a "flashy" oarsman, yet a good rower makes less commotion and senses a pick-up in boat speed. His propulsion efficiency is greater.

An example of reducing the puddle-loss energy is shown by non-feathering oars having a definite and repeatable blade entry angle downward, such as the 2 degree "dig" in figure 8. The blade easily and cleanly descends and rises through the water in the modified horizontal-plus-doryman's stroke. If these oars become inadvertently switched to the wrong side of the boat, the plus 2 degree dig becomes minus 2 degree, or 4 degree different than it should be. The blade doesn't descend easily, cavitates, and splashes more when entering and leaving the water. It pulls with a "washed out" feel, showing there is more slip and that it merely pushes the same water sternward with more kinetic energy loss, and so the boat loses its zip. When the oars are shifted to their correct sides, they bite more solidly on the descending catch and subsequent rise in "new" undisturbed water, and the puddle loss lessens.

Sometimes a boat feels like it is going "in the groove" on the instant of a firm catch when the oars have a fast, early bite with very little splashing, and the rower's rhythm is smooth and perfectly matches the boat speed at the moment. The trick of easy rowing is to stay "in the groove," even when the water gets rough and upsets that rhythm's precision, or when the rower is tired.

{16}

Selection of Oars

Some folks, thinking of rowing for the first time, ask how long oars should be, and they hear some arbitrary rule such as length should be twice the boat's beam, or the overlap should be 6", or the oars should just lack overlapping. While these rules may just happen to fit somebody in his particular boat, they won't fit all rowers and all boats, particularly the narrow boats. Six-foot oars for a 36" beam guide boat would require such a fast stroke that the rower couldn't keep up with himself, but 8-foot oars will turn the trick. As another example, the six different sizes of tuned oars (#1, 8, 31, 36, 37, and 43) in Table 1, ranging from 6'-6" to 9'long, show the futility of any rule-of-thumb selection because <u>all of these oars are usable by different people on the same boat but under different running conditions</u>. So there isn't much value in such rules. It is worth repeating that oar dimensions should not be forced to fit a boat except within very narrow limits. It is the oar's propulsive function to fit the rower to the boat's speed conditions. It is the separate function of the lock spread and overlap, if any, to dimensionally connect the oars to the boat and rower. The reason the above rules don't work is because there is no allowance for the rower's pull on the grip.

Picking oars is a trial and error procedure that has to start somewhere. One shortcut is to get into somebody else's boat, similar to the one you have in mind, and try different oars. If that is impossible, start with an oar traditional with that boat, even though most traditional oars can be improved. After becoming used to the first pair, you may want different ones and might analyze what to do in the light of this or other information.

Once the oars and rower are tuned up it becomes more fun to

row, particularly if the boat is easily moved and capable of long rows. Then it will be found that those first oars work best under certain running conditions and depending on the rower's energy level. If other running conditions appeal to the rower, he might consider taking along an additional pair of different oars to swap according to circumstances, or he may want more efficient oars.

The really interesting part about oars is designing and making your own. It is experimental work pure and simple, and is not difficult. In the following example, let's assume that the reader already has an easy-pulling pair for upwind work and wants a harder-pulling pair for calm or downwind rowing. If the requirement is the other way around, just move in the opposite direction. You can guess the dimensions for the new pair or try an almost rational approach, using the pull and work numbers, Y and WN.

The following simplified method treats an oar as a force lever pivoted at a definite lock location on the oar. A hand on the grip opposes a water force applied at the center of pressure (C.P.) on the blade. The oar is thwartwise, sweeping in a horizontal plane. The method also accounts for the work an oar does. Simplifying assumptions help practical solutions which are accurate enough for pleasure rowing. The method employs a combination of judgement and the use of numbers to design an oar.

The suggested design steps start with an existing oar as an example.

1. Measure dimensions A, B, BL, & W defined on Table 1, and enter them in column 2 of tabulation figure 10. The performance calculations are easily done working down the column using the formulae of Table 1, or by the chart figure 11

and the efficiency figures 6 or 7.

2. Decide the objective of designing new oars. Is it better downwind performance or a more suitable pull number for the regular oars, better efficiency, or a more powerful oar with a higher work number? This requires the designer to choose the pull number for the new oar, whether to change the pull number in column 2 for column 3. This is one bridge between columns 2 and 3. Figure 12 outlines possible initial assumptions for Y. Let's say the user finds his regular oars pull too easily downwind, hence his stroke rate is too high for comfort. This indicates a bigger downwind oar. So enter Y=21 for the new oar in column 3, figure 10. Then he would carry two pairs of oars. Table 1 has only one example of a downwind oar, number 31.

3. Let's try 7" blade width of the new oar and enter it in column 3, figure 10, realizing that the wider the blade, the shorter it is, the greater the propulsion efficiency, and the shorter the overall length, A.

4. Since blade length is related to it's width, the designer can either sketch a new blade with ample area of about 130 square inch, (since the blade can act as a sail downwind and shouldn't be feathered), or use figure 13 with about 2" added to the tip. Enter BL=23.5" on column 3, figure 10, and blade area=128 square inch.

5. Set inner loom length B. Avoid B under 24" and preferably get it up to 26" to 27". Let's enter B=25.5" in column 3, figure 10. B should be long

enough, because it is one determinant of work, WN. Obviously, the longer the handle end of a lever is, the more work can be done with the other end. Here WN=Y(B-2"). So the other determinant of WN is the pull number. At this design stage, check WN=21(25.5-2)=494, which looks reasonable. If WN looks too small and Y cannot be increased, then the only alternative is to increase B.

6. A handy formula shown on figure 12 is derived from the basic equations in Table 1. A=B+Y(B-2")/W+BL/5. It relates the important pull number to the oar dimensions. Each term on the right is a key oar length, adding up to total length, A. BL/5 was previously stipulated as an approximation, for the location of center of pressure in the derivation of the pull number Y in <u>Leverage</u> (section 11) and figure 3.

7. Now put the numbers that have been assembled in column 3, figure 10 into this formula:

   A=25.5+21(25.5-2)/7+4.7=101"=8′-5"

8. Find the base oar efficiency from the formulae on Table 1 or figure 6 or 7, and enter in column 3, figure 10. 73% looks good.

9. Grip overlap from the assumed lock spread of 46" is (2x25.5)-46=5", which is quite manageable. See <u>Overlap</u> (section 8). Since these are downwind oars, they work better not feathered. And the overlap manages easier without feathering.

10. Now compare columns 2 and 3 of figure 10 to see

if the new oar makes sense to do what is wanted. If not try another combination of assumptions.

11. After finishing a design, add 2" to the tip for good measure in case later adjusting is needed. If the oar pulls too hard do not cut more than 1" from the tip at a time, and be careful not to make the blade area too small.

12. If an oar pulls too hard there are several ways to reduce the pull number beside cropping the tip. In descending order of preference they are:

    a. Move the button outward on the oar to get longer inner loom and shorter outer loom for more leverage. Leave the blade alone.

    b. Shorten the oar by moving the button outward on the oar, and cutting off an equal length from the grip end. Leave the blade alone.

    c. Make the blade narrower, maybe a quarter inch at a time. The pull number is proportional to blade width. However, this also reduces blade area and efficiency, because the slip is increased.

    d. Be wary of any scheme that increases slip.

13. Always make the oar numbers before changing anything. It will save time and materials in the long run.

In summary, there are two general uses for the oar numbers. One is to find the performance characteristics of existing oars from their measurements (see column 2 of figure 10).

This is useful in comparing existing oars to find the best pull number for a rower. The other use given in column 3, figure 10, is designing new oars from scratch from certain given dimensions and a specified pull number. Of the several performance characteristics, the pull number is most important since it must be within the rower's capability, which varies widely between rowers and conditions. Also, if a rower determines his own charactristics, he will have a good design basis for his own customized oars.

It is not a good idea to only take the big oars out, leaving the regular oars home. I did that just once. A strong head wind suddenly sprang up and almost pulled my arms out of their sockets after about an hour of it, because when the head wind rises, the pull rises as the boat speed drops and the propulsion efficiency drops. It was like rowing against a dragging anchor.

A long-distance rowing race under varied conditions such as the Blackburn challenge race, would be a great opportunity for a fixed-seat rowboat to carry two pairs of oars with different pull numbers for each rower, if the rules allowed. The skillful use of two pairs of oars should significantly lower the rowing time, depending on how much conditions vary.

The blade offsets in figure 13 can be used as a starter when laying out the blade template, then modify according to your fancy. Try to maintain width near the center of water pressure because this is the best part of the blade considering both efficiency and drive. If it is a spoon blade, retain the tip width.

A 10% change in pull number from the existing oars to the new ones is about as small as can be felt and ordinarily

wouldn't justify making a new pair unless it is to be more efficient. The pull numbers of my two pairs of cruising oars are 16.8 and 22.8, which is a wide range of 1.36 to 1.0, and they act that way. Remember that in comparing two different oars with the same Q value, the oar with the higher work number will have the higher base oar efficiency (see figure 7).

The various graphs may show either or both of the two pairs of oars in Table 1, #43 for windward work and #31B for calms and downwind. Both of these oars can be improved upon, and they are not intended to be at the limits of the graphs. They are used in an easy-running, light boat, and their characteristics may be of some comparative use to others.

There is one simplification that runs through this whole story where numbers are concerned, and that is an omission of any attempt to calculate actual water forces on the blade. Such calculations, along with those of hull resistance under different wind and water conditions, the rower's energy, and the efficiencies, would be needed to find the equilibrium boat speed for a given stroke rate. Attempting these complex calculations would lessen the utility of this tale. As long as the stated limitations and assumptions of the methods given here are followed, there is a great deal of information to provide insight into the feel and water action of oars and possibly improve their breeds. Particularly is this the case on a long row when a nice breeze springs up astern and the big oars are used.

For those rowers interested in how the other fellow's oars compare, the pull, work, and base oar efficiency numbers can be obtained from the four basic oar dimensions A, B, BL, and W, with the owner's consent.

{17}

Pleasure Oar Improvements

Wouldn't an adjustable oar be great, one that suited all running conditions of the boat and rower? Theoretically, telescoping inner and outer looms would turn the trick, but practically, they would be hard to make and expensive. The same holds true with adjustable blades. Limited loom adjustments are possible with certain oars.

Some strong rowers can hold a feathering oar at a given point on a long buttonless leather to get the pull intensity they want, and they are unconcerned about imbalance. But many light rowers cannot do this and need a button. An adjustable button secured with an auto hose clamp or one that clamps on in halves works fine, although the counterweighting needs a solution; possibly a fixed counterweight for the outer button position and an additional one for the inner position. Buttons work for swivel yoke locks but not well for double thole pins. The flaws in this idea are that overlap might change too much and the greater work obtainable with a longer outer loom cannot be gotten into the shorter inner loom at the same time, unless a grip extension can be slipped over the handle, something I've never seen. However, the oar can be given a limited degree of harder or easier pull by moving the button or having double buttons spaced 3" to 4" apart.

The same idea might be used on a non-feathering North River style lock, such as the guide boat has, by boring several holes two inches apart in the oar and using a quick-change toggle pin. However, these schemes won't provide a big change in pull and work number unless a grip extension is used. My way to get more change is to take along two different pairs of oars.

A good Adirondack guide-boat oar is a tough one to improve, since the outer loom and blade usually are already shaved to the limit of light weight for the "carry." Nevertheless, most of these hardwood oars are blade heavy, particularly the eight footers, and they need counterbalancing. One possibility lies in the rectangular-octagonal inner loom which has more weight than strength requires. If the excess wood is removed so the loom is tapered and oval shaped for strength and minimum weight, then the counterweighting equivalent of the removed wood can be replaced with a *lesser* weight of lead within or near the grip, because the lead is farther from the lock than the removed wood. This will *lighten* the oar for the carry and lessen knuckle and knee interference. Oars which are not usually used for a carry can have counterweights added to the loom next to the grip, which I have done for a friend.

The inner and outer loom cross-sections of the non-feathering guide-boat oar are often higher than the width. This is contrary to the best distribution of wood for a minimum weight for a given bending strength in the direction of major pull. The reasons for this geometry are: *First*, the sawmill cuts the oar plank with a tapering thickness (thin end at blade tip) by canting the log between cuts; *Second*, the oars are very limber in the direction of pull, but not so much vertically, so their cross-sections are thinner horizontally than vertically. Also the oar needs some vertical stiffness to withstand the vertical slicing motion of the doryman's stroke, down then up. Perhaps these looms could be designed as limber single-leaf wooden springs, more later on guide-boat oars in *Very Limber Oars* (section 24).

I've seen several attempts to make spruce oars for guide boats, but the traditional yokes are too narrow to get a strong oar. Otherwise Sitka spruce is an ideal oar wood.

Characteristically, most old guide boats were made with local woods. So oak is never seen in the hull and Sitka spruce is absent in the oars.

Spoon oars with wide, short blades should improve the speed of traditional boats (or allow them to move with less energy) which customarily used oars with long, narrow, flat blades. See Oar Efficiency (section 14). But spoons require the rower to sit farther aft than for straight blades, see figure 5, and this isn't feasible with very high overlap grips, which require the rower to sit farther forward. This is the case with guide boats in their native Adirondacks. Also, racers and non-racers there must preserve the traditional look or be disqualified and even ostracized. An outrigger lock, even a folding one, would be an encumbrance and hazardous complexity in the deep Adirondack woods and narrow brooks.

However, oars in the Adirondacks might be made with somewhat wider and shorter straight blades, still remain within the traditional look, and have higher propulsion efficiency. Guide boats elsewhere in open water might use folding locks to reduce overlap so feathering or non-feathering spoons could be used. Thus equipped, a guide boat (still fixed-seat) ought to get around very well indeed. Good spoons in a fast boat, my what a pleasure that is!

With suitable lock span, other narrow craft such as the St. Lawrence skiff can be fitted with higher-efficiency spoon oars. Many coastal craft readily take spoons because they are beamier and don't have overlap, or very little.

Incidentally, I don't apologize for frequently mentioning the Adirondack guide boat (no, I don't own one) because it provides many good examples, transports easily, is very

responsive, and makes a superb traditional wooden racing boat among its other general uses. It does require excellent care and seamanship. It is impossible for a sporty rower to avoid turning up the main burner at times to blow off the dust. There is enough variety among guide boats so that some of them are naturally better suited for specific purposes than others. The only traditional fixed-seat rowboat that can beat a guide boat is another one. The most accurate and detailed guide boat plans published are for the type built by D. Grant, drawn by John Gardner, and described by him in his chapter in The Adirondack Guide Boat by K. and H. Durant (Camden: International Marine Publishing, 1980). He also includes detailed dimensions for Grant soft maple oars with the following characteristics according to the notation of these articles: A=96"; B=24"; BL=24"; W=5+3/8"; Y=16.4; WN=360; (BE)=71%. These figures compare well with other guide-boat oars.

Copper-tipped blades eventually crack at the rivets, and the usual rounded corners lose part of the most effective blade area. Copper tips are usually thicker at the end than necessary, and they lack the sharp edge to inhibit water flow around the end. Therefore they will slip easier. Pre-formed copper tips aren't wide enough for efficient blades. In these respects, a thin, square-cornered tip encased in fiberglass is superior and more durable, but admittedly less handsome than a glued wooden inlay, which must necessarily be thicker for strength, and be used carefully or not at all on rocks. Such a glass tip can be neatly made, although it will mortify a pure traditionalist. See figure 13.

Feathering oars with experimental leathers of du Pont Teflon are being tried. Teflon, with its remarkably low coefficient of dry friction against a polished bronze

swivel-yoke lock, requires mimimal feathering effort. The oars feel as if mounted on ball bearings. Teflon is waterproof, corrosion resistant, and available in sheets 1/16" thick and more. Thus far it shows no scuffing after 3-1/2 years. The lock must be well polished and have no sharp corners or ridges contacting the Teflon. A button is required as otherwise the Teflon is so slippery that it is almost impossible to hold the oar in one spot endwise in the lock. If the button is put on over the Teflon, extra pains must be taken to secure the button because it will slide easily too. Teflon's further advantage is that it needn't be slathered with lubricant. This is nice if clean sails and the like are aboard. Teflon washers, 1-1/2" diameter, used under non-feathering oars slipped over single thole pins, work better than leather.

The slot-hole leathers of the non-feathering St. Lawrence skiff oar have a combination rolling and sliding motion against the single thole pin, particularly the after leather bearing against the pin on the pull. Most leathers will bunch up ahead of the pin causing added friction even when lubricated (analogous to pedalling a bicycle in deep sand). By substituting the harder dry surface and far less friction of polyethylene cut from a milk jug for the after "leather" only, the pin friction is very much less. Then, with a Teflon washer under the oar, it moves so easily that the blade, if set to dig at the catch, will dive with less friction than real leather. The oar has more zip, and the rower has a keener feel of the blade action in the water. The polyethylene "leather" is harder to install as it must be warmed in hot water to roll half of it up to pass through the slot-hole in the oar. The nice thing about polyethylene is its ready availability. Keep real leather on the forward side of the slot-hole, because it sticks enough to prevent the oar from jumping the pin on a strong backing stroke.

Racing spoon oars have a flat on the forward side of the loom (when pulling) which engages a mating, flat sided horn of the swivel-yoke lock. This is essential for the feathering oar to get a consistent blade entry angle into the water where every stroke counts. Very few feathering pleasure oars have these worthwhile flats. The flats make the oars permanently right and left handed if the blades aren't set on the vertical when pulling. Wider feathering blades are more sensitive to the correct blade entry angle, so wide blades really need the flats. Flats, if too loose, can make a noisy, rattling feathering oar.

Straight blades with the working face flat or slightly concave and the opposite face crowned, should have a firmer grab on the water (should slip less) than blades of equal area crowned on both faces. I don't know how much the improvement would be.

If the oars attending a small craft convention are a fair sample of the whole oar population, untuned oars have an overwhelming vote. Although it takes about as long to tune oars as it does to make them before tuning, this is still a very practical thing to do with most existing oars.

Since wood varies, it is almost impossible to make a new tuned oar the first time exactly to the dimensions of a sketch. So sketch dimensions should be liberal in blade and outer loom thicknesses, and the oar roughed out to them. Then tune, first to get the desired spring, and then balance to the required P.

It is nice to start making a pair of oars with wood for both of equal intrinsic stiffness and density. But that is not absolutely necessary if tuning is done. I have tuned a pair wherein each oar was a different species of softwood,

having different density and modulus of elasticity (I doubt that a hardwood oar could be tuned satisfactorily against a softwood mate). After reaching the same measured spring in both oars there was a difference in the two outer loom thicknesses noticeable only when the oars were laid alongside each other. There was considerable difference in the amount of counterbalancing lead to give the same P balance, and quite a difference in the total weights. But, the locks bear the weight, and they don't complain. There was a difference in the inertia, F values, but it was of secondary importance, and the color was different. Otherwise the oars felt as if made of the same piece of wood.

If you break an oar that can't be fixed (almost impossible) and cannot find matching wood for a new oar, proceed anyway with the closest equivalent wood, and tune both oars to the same spring and P balance. One way to shorten the time needed to make oars is to convert old, long, spruce racing spoons to shorter, fixed-seat oars as was done with oars #43 in Table 1. Originally these 50-60 year olds were 9'-9" long. They were reworked using the ideas in this article. They have souped up my skiff, becoming my favorite oars. The characteristic numbers are about right for me for heavy going to windward in a smart boat. These oars also do well in lighter conditions. The changes were: 25" cut off the grip end; the inner blade ends were trimmed away 2" to reduce windage and backing of water when the water pivot point moves outward when the boat runs faster; the central rib of the spoon blade was removed to lessen splashing and turbulence in vertical blade movement; spruce blocks were glued to the outer loom at the new lock location; the slot-hole cut and leathered in traditional St. Lawrence skiff style; the blade angle was set to dig 4 degrees with the oar thwartwise; the outer loom was shaved to lighten it and provide spring; the blades needed extensive repair; the

copper tips were scrapped and the blade tips thinned down and neatly glassed; copper pennies (lead was lacking at the time) were stashed inside the big 1+3/4" diameter grips for balance, which cost a total of $1.27 U.S. and Canadian, plus leftover Spanish corks in the grip ends. These large straight grips have never produced any blisters. I definitely recommend the re-incarnation of expired racing sculls found in old garrets and boat sheds, for rejuvenating our prized fixed-seat relics among the traditional small craft, if the sculls are repairable and the spoon blades are wide enough to begin with.

The windage of non-feathering oars is sometimes a disadvantage in stiff going to windward. This is more pronounced with blades having excessive area, see Table 1. Substituting a wide, short-bladed, high-efficiency spoon oar with consequently less blade area will partly offset the windage. Good spoons would be very helpful for example, on the St. Lawrence River which is often pretty breezy.

{18}

Fitting the Rower to the Boat

Pleasure oars are only that when the rower is a natural fit to his oars, boat, and the sometimes rough water surface. The ideal is a rower who is an integral part of his surroundings, and he will be if his hands, feet, and rump are comfortable. Efficient rowing requires a minimum of energy lost in discomfort. So in addition to tuning our oars, lets tune up our boats.

Rigid dimensional rules might be made for the average-sized rower, but real comfort means tailoring the location of seats and stretcher with respect to the locks, oars, and water to suit each individual. This can be done sometimes with the boat and oars to be used. But when the boat was unavailable or in the design stage, a rowing mock-up out in the yard worked fine for me many years ago. Incidentally, one of my friends asked me later whether the neighbors expected to see me fishing in a pail of water too. The mock-up can consist of a footstool shimmed up to the right height to sit on, and with the cushion to be used, if any; a log for a stretcher, large enough in diameter so it will touch the balls of the rower's feet; and a stake in the ground for each oar lock with the height above ground equal to the depth of the boat at the lock, and the spread to mimic the lock span of the boat. Refer to <u>Inner Loom Length</u> (section 12).

For flat-bladed oars the fore-and-aft location of the seat and stretcher should allow the middle of the stroke, whether long or short, to coincide with the thwartwise oar position. For spoon oars the middle of the stroke would be better located if it came with the outer loom at an angle forward of thwartwise equal to the angle of the tip of the spoon with respect to the long oar axis (see figure 5). The

reason for this is seen in the slip diagrams, figures 1g and 1h, because the hook of the tip of the spoon will kick too much water inward toward the boat at the end of the stroke unless the whole stroke at the blade is advanced by sitting farther aft. As a sharp old timer said, "It's like putting on the brakes" if the spoon blades come out of the water too late.

The seat height should allow the oar grips to be held low without hitting the knees or thighs on the recovery in rough water with some heel of the boat. A little more grip clearance for rough water can be gained by removing the seat cushion. This has the added benefit of lowering the rower's weight to enhance the stability of a narrow-waterline boat in broken water.

Most stretchers have too coarse an adjustment, are too narrow, and too low to take advantage of the strong spring in one's foot which is an excellent shock absorber of oar thrust. The horizontal distance from the lock should fit the rower very closely. And the stretcher height in the middle should come up to the base of the toes. It should go far enough across the boat so the feet can wander along it to avoid cramping and make it easier for the rower to turn his head to pick his way among rocks. Also, feet spread apart are good balance sensors and steady the rower in the center of the boat in rough water. When the rower has to scratch for a precarious foothold with his heels or the sides of his feet against small rounded ribs, he wastes energy and cannot get a strong pull when the occasion demands. When the stretcher is in the right place the rower instantly becomes part of the boat when his foot touches it. The best stretcher is built in solidly, strengthens the boat, and fits only the owner and others like him.

The traditional guide boat is very unsatisfactory in

requiring the rower to dig with his heels against the copper-sheathed ribs crossing the bottom board at 5" to 6" intervals. However, those boats used for racing have been allowed in recent years to use stretchers which sometimes consist of a piece of old rake handle set across the boat in a fixed position to meet the ball of the foot. These stretchers are extremely effective. One weight-conscious guide-boat builder uses a bamboo stick built into his pleasure boat. Many other types of boats could follow this example for pleasure rowing. Personally, I row as much with my feet as with my hands even though the seat is fixed.

Once the mock-up is done, its dimensions can be transferred to the boat. However, the thwart should first be located in the boat to get the right fore-and-aft trim and then the locks and stretcher located to suit. To locate the rowing thwart, it is useful to know that the rower's c.g. is about at the navel.

Note that the rowing mock-up isn't used to design the oars as they already exist. Rather, it is used to find the best fit of the rower to his boat and oars so he can get the best performance out of himself and his equipment. Most rowboats, classic and otherwise, are a poor fit to many of us and we cannot get the best out of them. A rowing mock-up may also lead to a useful and unconventional seat arrangement, as it did for me.

{19}
Blade Buoyancy

An ideal balanced oar in most respects may still have too much blade buoyancy that interferes with getting a snappy, deep dig on the catch. There is a simple floatation test to detect excessive blade buoyancy in an oar balanced for a given person. With the boat in the water, the oar in its lock extending thwartwise, and no hand on the grip, note how much, if any, of the blade shoulder appears above water. If, say, less than about an inch appears, then the blade buoyancy isn't too much, and the buoyancy will not slow the dig of the oar into the water. Naturally, an oar that has to be forced deeper than its floating test level, is going to require more effort while submerged.

Oars made of denser woods, such as ash, soft maple, birch, and cherry, are very resilient to shock, and can have thinner blades, flexible yet strong. Since the volume of these thin blades is less, and the wood density is greater, they have relatively lower buoyancy and can dig well. However, oars of light, softwood, such as spruce, tend to have thicker blades to get enough strength. So the volume of these blades and their buoyancy is greater and may slow down a fast dig into the water at the catch. So, it is desirable to thin the blades as much as the type of wood will allow, before adding the counterweight. This applies to all oar woods.

While it is important to counterweight an oar so it balances with the blade out of water and with a hand on the grip, ideally, the blade should have no buoyancy, so the oar still feels balanced the same way when the blade is submerged. The nearest this ideal can be met is to minimize blade volume by having the blade as thin as possible, and have a blade area no greater than is needed for efficient

propulsion.

In Table 1, ash oar #8 is a dandy one, 57 years old. It has a thin, flexible blade. It is balanced and digs very well. Many hardwood guide-boat oars have thin flexible blades, some of them of very flexible soft maple. This applies particularly to oar #13, which was successfully used for racing for about 40 years.

Spruce oar #43 is balanced and digs well. In the above floatation test only about one inch of the blade shoulder is above water. So very little effort is needed to submerge the blade.

Spruce oar #31 has about 2-1/2" of shoulder above water, so it has too much blade buoyancy, and it feels that way. It doesn't dig well. This blade could be thinned more, which would also allow some counterweight to be removed.

Most commercial oars, as received, have blades too thick and buoyant. But, they can be readily improved by thinning.

Referring to the dig angle mentioned in Blade Area and Shape (section 15), and Balance (section 3), it is evident that there is a relation between balance, dig, blade buoyancy, blade strength, and the rower's physique. This is one of the facets of fun with oars.

{20}
Impulse

Oars are impulse tools to propel a rowboat with a periodic surging motion. And the details of impulse can supply insight into how oars work and what might be done to improve their design and usage. While this subject gets a bit technical, it will shortly shake down to some easily understood concepts that explain how oars act.

Physical impulse is a force multiplied by the duration of time the force is applied to move an object, Fxt. In our case the force applied to accelerate the boat forward during the pull is the residual force, F, of the oars after subtracting the water, wind, and chop resistance, if any, of the hull to forward motion. The lateral water forces on the oars cancel each other when using a pair of oars. Plot F vertically on a graph against time, t, horizontally. See figure 14, curve A, for one pull. The catch starts at t=0 and F=0. The pull ends when t=t1 and F is back to zero as the recovery begins. After the recovery the process repeats at the catch of the next stroke.

It turns out that the area enclosed under the curve is the total impulse of the pull and is proportional to the increase in momentum of the boat and contents during the pull. If we neglect the to-and-fro motion of the fixed-seat rower, then the total impulse area under the curve is proportional to the increase in boat velocity during the pull, and this surge is what we want. The proof of the foregoing is rather simple and is put in the appendix with figure 14. So here is a general concept that we can easily use without putting down actual numbers or drawing an accurate impulse curve, which would be very hard to do. We just use our imaginations to think of ways to get more impulse area under the curve for a given stroke rate. Bear

in mind during this discussion, that after a steady stroke rate is reached, the increase in boat velocity during the pull is balanced by a corresponding decrease during recovery.

Assume curve A is for a moderate pull with a flat blade moving primarily in horizontal sweeping motion where the blade is pushing through water part of the time, mostly near and at its thwartwise position, and slicing outward in the forestroke followed by slicing inward in the afterstroke, per figures 1c, 1g, and 1h in Slip (section 6). A wide spoon tip will be a better slicer in the forestroke, but not good in the afterstroke if carried too far aft. So make the forestroke longer and the afterstroke shorter in time to get the same total time. This will help fill out the impulse area in the left upper corner, as in curve B, and make the boat a little faster at the end of the pull with a spoon oar. And the spoon properties will affect the grab efficiency at the catch.

Note that in using the impulse diagram, we have to keep the idea of linear arc length of the pull separate from the idea of time duration of the pull, which is what the impulse curve area is based on.

If we pull harder, the flat blade curve A will rise, but the duration of the pull for a given arc of pull will be shorter because the slip is greater, so we haven't done much to get more impulse area per stroke. But if we lengthen the arc of the stroke a little along with the stronger pull, and lengthen the time duration of the pull, then the impulse area has increased to curve C. And that is usually how we would pick up boat speed.

We could go to oars with bigger blades to match the stronger pull for the same length of time as curve A, and

result in curve D with greater impulse area than for curve A. This is where more powerful rowers can use wider blades or longer oars with higher pull and work numbers for a given stroke rate and go faster, or row easier for a given speed, than the weaker rowers. (See pull number Y defined in Leverage (section 11) and work number WN defined in Inner Loom Length (section 12).

The impulse diagram can be used to show the effect of entrained air on the forward face of the blade. Because the blade suddenly drops out of air into water at the catch, there is always the possibility of trapping some air on the forward blade face. How much air is trapped makes a difference on how hard the oar pulls.

In a simplified concept for a totally submerged flat blade moving perpendicularly to water, the pressure face has a drag coefficient of 1.0, and the suction face has a coefficient of 0.8, for a total of 1.8. If the suction face is entirely covered by an air pocket, its drag coefficient is about 0.0 which yields a total coefficient of only 1.0. So the pull on the oar for comparable velocity of the blade against water would only be 1.0/1.8=56% of the pull for a blade with no air pocket. The air gives an oar a "washed out" feel (see curve E). In this case the impulse area is very low because both the force, F, is low and the time duration is short. So there is only a feeble increase in boat velocity during the pull. With amounts of entrained air between the above limits, the total drag coefficient will vary between 1.8 and 1.0. So it is up to the rower to use the oar in a manner to avoid the entrained air by keeping the blade submerged enough and at a dig angle to wipe off the air as the blade enters the water. The details of blade cross-section may also affect entrainment of air.

The rower may get a momentary glimpse of the entrained air,

if any, when visibility conditions are good if the water is clear and calm, and the sun is bright and overhead. Then sometimes the air, if a small amount, can be seen in a trailing vortex off the tip of the blade right after the catch. This is a poor man's simple video camera of tip vortices for oar research.

Now comes the interesting part. If vertical slicing action of the oar through the water, down after the catch and up before the release in the doryman's stroke, figure 9, is added to the horizontal sweeping motion of the oar, as well as slices outward and inward, there is added hydrodynamic thrust forward in both the upper corners of the impulse graph as in curve F. This increases the impulse area and results in greater surge in boat speed during the pull. Adjusting the dig angle to get the most benefit from the doryman's stroke is part of the final tuning of an oar and it is very effective in improving the grab of the blade at the catch. The impulse diagram shows why.

I suspect the greatest potential improvement in the future in oars for our traditional fixed-seat pleasure boats lies in the doryman's stroke portion when combined with the sweeping motion. Here the three-dimensional geometry of the blade has to be related to the rower's motion pattern of how deep and fast the blade descends and later ascends, and how long and fast the deep blade will travel horizontally when near thwartwise.

For the vertical motion the blade is much like a hydrofoil, which will have some optimum cross-section and attack angle to give maximum hydrodynamic "lift" forward. But, unlike most applications of aero-hydrodynamic theory, the oar blade is surrounded by a host of transient flows and forces (same for the rowboat's forward motion through water). So the best we can do as individuals who are unlikely to have

sophisticated test equipment, is to use steady flow theory and experiment with blade shapes by cut and try methods. For this the book of C.A. Marchaj, Aero-hydrodynamics of Sailing is a good source of information on lift coefficients and attack angles of some foil sections that might be practical for reversible blades, moving down then up. Note that there is nothing specific in this book about oars. We have to apply the data with imagination.

A similar but very professional attempt has been under way to improve Olympic kayak paddles with foil cross-sections for a slicing motion through the water superposed on the dragging motion. These have been called "wing blades" and they require a different muscle structure of the paddler. As pleasure rowers we don't have to go that far, but giving oar blades a foil section for the doryman's stroke is within our physical capability (see Washington Post, 29 April 1990, B-14).

Most of our traditional fixed-seat rowboats and those derived from them have enough initial lateral stability for the doryman's deep slicing stroke. And the more the stability, the stronger the dig can be. This is impossible with the narrow sliding-seat boats lest they upset. Their oars have what they call positive blade pitch, or what I would call negative dig angle, in order to prevent the blades from digging more on one side than the other and capsizing. So they really cannot exploit the doryman's stroke and utilize the possible forward hydrodynamic "lift" of a descending and ascending blade. This will be up to us fixed-seaters.

The annual Howard Blackburn rowing and paddling races around Cape Ann are a real challenge to develop better oars, paddles, and boats in all kinds of conditions from quiet to very rough. It will be interesting to keep an eye

on these race results if the races continue over a period of years. They attract good rowers and paddlers in a marvelous laboratory of experience. And there should eventually be some benefit for pleasure craft also.

The elements of force and time in impulse can be remembered readily if we visualize Father Isaac Newton, aided by Father Time, in pushing Father Neptune along in his light cockleshell with an intermittent surge. Naturally, this famous trio is singing the songs of the old voyageurs in the Canadian fur trade, swinging the paddles of their ancient bateaux and canoes in musical unison.

{21}

Grab at the Catch

A firm, quick grab is a dandy way to start a high impulse stroke to kick a rowboat along. The rower can largely control the speed of blade descent, and if it is a feathering oar with a round loom at the lock, he can roughly control the dig angle. However, this is difficult to do consistently and accurately for most pleasure rowers. There are also several design features that can help get a fast and strong grab, and these are among the key parts of tuning an oar.

1. Thin the blade for minimum buoyancy, which otherwise tends to delay the blade descent in the water.

2. Thin the blade consistent with strength to get minimum blade weight. Also thin the outer loom likewise with an elliptical cross section with major axis in pull direction. (Note the exception for very limber oars in <u>Pleasure Oar Improvements</u> (section 17)). This weight reduction also reduces the amount of counterweight, if any, all of which lessens the inertia of the oar to allow the blade to drop into the water as fast as possible. In this respect a lively oar is a real pleasure to use. The rower should be able to feel the water action on the blade, not the inertia of an unwieldy oar.

3. Thin the blade, including the edges, so there will be minimum fuss when the blade is forcefully driven into the water with the least chance of entraining air, which softens the pull and lowers impulse.

4. Keep the blade cross section a clean foil design free from ridges or loom extensions down the middle of either face. Here we want to use the blade in the doryman's stroke. Remember, airplane wings haven't gotten around to ridges extending outward along the middle of either upper or lower surfaces. Try a blade cross-section with a flat or concave after face and a crowned forward face to get more "lift" forward (see Marchaj, _Aero-hydrodynamics of Sailing_).

5. Use a lock that will give accurate and repeatable control of dig angle of blade into the water. The lift of a foil can be sensitive to the angle of attack as the steep curves in Marchaj, page 319, show. More on this in the next topic.

6. Have the pull on the oar help the blade descend.

The reason for the need of a very fast grab is that prior to the fully-developed pull the external forces on the boat of hull resistance, and often wind and chop resistance, are slowing it down. These forces have to be first overcome by the forward force of the water against the blade _before_ acceleration of the boat commences. And then the acceleration will take time to build up to full effectiveness. Yet the blade should be quickly and cleanly submerged in moving water with no entrained air _before_ the pull starts. To do all this it takes time from the instant the blade starts to reverse its path coming out of the recovery until the acceleration of the boat is developed. During this time the boat is slowing down, the oar is losing part of its stroke arc and impulse time, and a lot has to happen. The blade and rower's arm and body motions are following a complicated path and building up the pull

to suit sea, wind, and speed conditions required. This split second is when the rower's practiced skill and coordination are in greatest demand. This is the moment when getting the boat "in the groove" starts, alluded to in Blade Area and Shape (section 15), last paragraph. It is the moment of magic conspiracy when the well-tuned rower pulls a perfectly tuned oar in a tuned rowboat. Automatic precision of the reflexes are the catch words.

{22}

Blade Dig Angle

A strong grab at the catch as well as the forward hydrodynamic "lift" of a blade in the doryman's stroke depends on the actual or true dig angle, T.D.A., of the blade into the water. There are really three other angles involved, and T.D.A. is the resultant of all three.

1. The oar itself may be made with the blade at a different angle from the lock in the non-feathering oar or from the angle at the flat on a feathering oar which bears against a straight forward horn of a swivelling lock.

2. The lock may have an outward cant angle. This is found in many non-feathering St. Lawrence skiff single thole pins and on some non-feathering locks with a horizontal pin running through the oar and both horns of a swivel yoke lock. The Adirondack guide-boat lock is this type, although most of the guide boats I have seen have vertical stems. So lock cant angle is not a factor for them.

3. There is a swing angle of the oar forward and aft of thwartwise which affects T.D.A. for those blades with canted locks.

Combining these three angles to get the T.D.A. at any position during the stroke is a trigonometric exercise done in the appendix, figure 15, using the single thole pin lock of the St. Lawrence skiff as an example with the results shown on figure 16, which apply to all canted lock types where the cant angle affects T.D.A. Several actual examples are shown on figure 16 by tracing the arrows. Any pin cant angle outward will adversely affect dig at the catch.

A convenient rule of thumb for outward-canted locks is that for a catch at 40 degrees swing angle from thwartwise, the reduction in dig angle is 2/3 of the outward cant angle. For example, a blade having a built-in dig angle of 3 degrees on a lock canted outward 6 degrees, the T.D.A. at catch will be 3-(2/3x6)=minus 1 degree, which could be far from what the rower expected from a 3-degrees-dig blade angle. For one thing the air might not wipe off as fast at the catch. All this complication can be avoided by setting the locks vertical.

The feathering oar without a flat in the plain swivel yoke commonly seen also has its dig angle adversely affected at the catch if the yoke stem cants outward unless the rower turns the oar in the lock during the pull, which isn't easily done with the precision that the best attack angle of a foil cross-section of a blade seems to require. So for these oars a flat is suggested with a vertical stem lock.

If it is desired to increase T.D.A. of a blade throughout the pull, the lock can be canted outward and the oar given more of its own compensating dig angle to give the proper T.D.A. at the catch. Likewise, if it is desired to decrease the T.D.A. during the pull, the lock should be canted inward, all as shown on figure 16.

As mentioned previously, digging oars are never used in low or zero-stability, narrow sliding-seat boats, but they are fine for the stabler fixed-seat boats using the doryman's stroke. Adirondack guide boats are tiddly. Their oars do not dig. Whether this is the result of unsuccessful experience with digging oars or whether as a practical matter the oars should be interchangeable side to side, I do not know. The answer to my question has always been, "that's the way it has always been done." Once a digging

style oar is chosen it is not interchangeable with the oar on the other side. Nothing serious is likely to happen if crossed. Instead of a nice grab at the catch there might be a negative dig with the oar sucking air and there would be a "wash out" pull, all immediately detected on the first pull. A negative-dig oar might tend to jump the lock on a strong pull. If you break a digging oar it should be replaced with a similar oar.

While so far I have had no stability problem with 4-degrees-dig spoon oars in a lightweight, modified St. Lawrence skiff (75 lbs.), I don't know how much more than 4 degrees, it will tolerate in rough water.

In all of the above, when a vertical lock is mentioned, functionally the vertical lock axis should be perpendicular to the water surface at the blades. Practically, this is setting the lock perpendicular to the waterline plane of the boat, which would be a rough average of the water level at the blades in broken water.

Getting a good grab with the proper lock setting and true dig angle of the blade into the water at the catch is part of tuning the boat as well as the oar.

{23}

Rowboat Surging

As each pull of the oars produces a surge in the boat's forward motion, the surge strength at a particular moment is defined by the boat's forward acceleration at that moment. Here Isaac Newton and his second law of motion are conjured up once more. F=(W/g)xa, where F is lbs. force applied to an object of weight, W lbs., g is gravitational constant 32.2 ft./sec squared, and a is the object's (boat's) acceleration ft/sec. squared. This is rewritten a=(g/W)xF. In our case F is the residual accelerating forward force on the boat at any instant after subtracting water, wind, and chop resistance forces RW, RB, and RC respectively, which hold the boat back. If FT is the total forward push of the oars on the boat, then F=FT-RW-RB-RC and the acceleration expression is a=(g/W)x(FT-RW-RB-RC). RW is always with us if the boat is in motion, RB and RC are present if there is wind or chop. This expression agrees with the obvious experience that the stronger the pull on the oars, and the smaller the resistances are, and the lighter the boat (W is in the denominator), the greater the acceleration will be. Note that RW, RB, and RC are speed dependant. The faster the boat goes, the more the resistances slow it down and partially counteract an increased pull, FT. So not all of the benefit of greater pull is realized to accelerate the boat. FT is affected by the design and use of the oars. The resistances are governed by the design of the boat to suit conditions to be encountered.

It turns out very neatly that the ordinate, F, of the impulse curve, figure 14, at any instant is also the force F in the above surge expression. So the nature of the impulse curve is affected by acceleration. A smooth horizontal-sweeping stroke will likely have a single hump

in the impulse curve about near the middle and at the top of which the maximum acceleration will occur. A vigorous doryman's stroke will have an impulse curve with two humps, each denoting a surge with its own acceleration, and two surges per pull.

It is peculiar that the rower doesn't feel the surge he produces in the boat, because his body is in motion. But a passenger seated quietly can feel the acceleration of the surge if it is strong enough, because his body wants to stay behind when the boat surges forward. Actually, it is the passenger's response to the acceleration of two surges on a single pull that allows us to infer that the impulse curve has two humps corresponding to the doryman's stroke on a vigorous pull. If the stroke is not strong, the passenger may feel only one surge. Admittedly, this is a very subjective test and will not detect weak surges that may be present. But it is a simple test for a knowledgeable passenger to make in a light boat with a strong rower.

Some of the surge energy is absorbed on board by the motion of anything that moves, such as the swaying of a passenger, swashing of bilge water, if any, or even water in a bait pail. Probably most of the surge energy will be absorbed outside the boat by a surge in the bow wave and a sudden increase in skin friction loss. A very sudden surge may cause a momentary cresting of the bow wave. Water, even though deformable, does not like to be moved aside fast, and the faster and the more of it that is diverted, the more solid its resistance. Water can be as hard as concrete if disturbed fast enough. Light boats tend to surge a lot as explained previously, so they dissipate more energy, which robs them of speed. The way to reduce this loss is to design the boat with sharper water lines and less displacement at and near the bow and reduce wetted surface. This is also the way to design for lower bow wave loss in a

chop. The modern sea kayak is a good example.

The rowboats with a double surge on one pull seem to fall in a class by themselves. They are among the lightest boats and are propelled by the doryman's stroke with its additional hydrodynamic "lift" on the down and up slices. Among these double surgers are the Adirondack guide boat, a light St. Lawrence skiff (75 lbs.), and a light Irish curragh, all when driven hard. I have felt the double surge in the first two of the above boats when the rower plunged his oars down at the catch and yanked them up before the release. It was the addition of the strong vertical blade motion to the horizontal sweeping motion that made the surges so prominent. The guide-boat oars were like #13 in Table 1. The blades were thin with thin edges, very limber, with a slight smooth crown on both faces, no ridge on either side, and non-feathering. It was a racing-stroke rate probably about 55 per minute, which with the double surge made about 110 surges per minute, very favorable for speed in a light boat. The dig angle was exactly the same for every stroke as it had been for many years, impossible to do with the ordinary feathering oar at that high stroke rate.

The curragh oar has a deceptively ungainly look at a cursory glance, but it sure works. I measured a set of these oars for a 23-foot, three-man, Boston (Dorchester) planked curragh with blades shown in figure 17. While these particular oars were only 8 feet long, compared to 10 to 11 feet or more for oars in Western Ireland, with about 2-1/4"-wide blades, their use is about the same with the doryman's stroke. These oars are not efficient if used in a shallow sweeping horizontal stroke because the long narrow blades have so much slip at the tip which results in high turbulence loss in the water. However, if given the doryman's deep stroke their long blade has high vertical

slicing velocity and consequently a strong "lift" forward with a double impulse matching the down and up stroke motion. Note that the Boston blade has a better foil cross-section than a plain rectangular section which appears to be the case elsewhere. The after face of the Boston oar is flat and the forward face is crowned. There would probably be a little better "lift" forward for the vertical motion if the after face was slightly cupped (see Marchaj, Aero-hydrodynamics of Sailing, page 319).

There may be other types of noticeably double-surging traditional fixed-seat rowboats that I don't know about. If so, I suspect they are light and also use essentially the doryman's stroke. The curragh, like the guide boat is a very sporty racing boat when driven by a high-spirited crew. An advantage of the long, narrow curragh blades in vertical slicing motion through the water is their high aspect ratio, which tends toward high efficiency. And even though the blades are in transient water flow, the circulation flow around their cross section, on which forward lift depends, is more quickly established for foils with short chords. The vertical blade motion is pivoted about the lock whereas for the horizontal sweeping motion the pivot point functionally is at the water pivot point usually near the blade neck of an ordinary oar (see Slip, section 6). So, comparatively, the long length of the curragh oar from lock to tip, and the deep slice, help attain high vertical speed of the tip through the water, which enhances the forward "lift" there. So for both motions the tip region of the blade is the most effective in driving the boat.

It appears that whenever we see an indigenous long, narrow blade for an oar or paddle used in some part of the world, we are looking at a blade intended to be sliced as well as pushed through the water, and that the blade was probably

developed long before formal hydrodynamics was invented. So blade shape is a possible clue to how the blade is used.

Two ways to reduce the surge losses for an existing light boat and improve its performance are to increase stroke rate so the boat doesn't slow down so much between pulls and also maintains a higher propulsion efficiency, and to use very limber oars.

When designing a new light rowboat for speed (and consequently easy rowing) where surging motion from the oars will be active, I haven't found useable data. Tank and full-size towing tests seem to be restricted to constant speed in calm water, which I believe does not suit the wide variety of actual conditions. I suspect longer forward lines favor lower surge and chop resistance. So rowboat design is still "seat of the pants," which is most interesting.

One of the secrets of lightweight, easy-rowing boat design is preventing the boat velocity during recovery from excessively slowing down due to hull resistance and adverse sea and wind conditions. The Eskimo's hunting kayak is a fine example of an ancient design going to the heart of intermittent propulsion. And high-stroke-rate oars or paddles shorten the most critical time while the craft is coasting with decaying velocity.

To try adapting a good heavy rowboat to light construction, in order to reduce displacement and thereby attempt to increase its speed, may not be as effective an approach as also altering the lines so there is less resistance with an easier hull shape.

{24}

Very Limber Oars

This is a later contination of the earlier discussion of Stiffness (section 5). Another functional similarity between Adirondack guide-boat and curragh oars is their great limberness, which must have developed by far different routes. When the Adirondack folks are asked why the guide-boat oars are so limber the usual answer is they have always been that way. Those who developed the limber oar are long gone, so we are unlikely to get firsthand accounts. And the curragh oar is far older, the lock at least, going back to the Phoenicians.

Aside from the differences in availability of good oar wood, the necessity to carry light oars on a portage, and the great difference in usage of oars on a wide, rough sea, or on lakes and narrow streams, these boats are alike in having a sharp double surge that is softened with a limber oar, which transfers impulse area from under the first part of the impulse curve of figure 14 to a later part, retaining the area intact.

Even though the guide boat has sharp lines forward, the bow wave loss must be greater the more sudden the surge. Movies show this definite bow wave surge. Both boats when not loaded are light enough compared to the human power in them to accelerate very quickly at the catch when the first surge occurs. If their oars were not limber, there would be a more sudden surge. But since the oars bend so much, they absorb some of the rower's energy at the catch, and there is a momentary softening or delay of the surge of the boat which must be reflected in less energy loss in the bow wave and other surge losses.

Also, the limberness delays the acceleration of blade slip

through the water and reduces the turbulent energy losses around the blade in the puddle, all of which conserves more of the rower's energy to drive the boat in lower parts of the impulse curve. In effect, the boat feels a smoother stroke from the rower. The very limber oar also reduces the surge losses of the boat at the catch, because it allows the rower's upper body to move farther forward than he would with a stiffer oar. By the law of conservation of momentum this extra forward momentum of the rower's body must be compensated by a simultaneous equal reduction in forward momentum of the boat. So the boat's forward acceleration is reduced at the catch with an accompanying lower surge loss in the bow wave and in any other surge losses. Again, the lighter the boat with its greater accelerating tendency, the more effective very limber oars are. This applies to both guide boats and curraghs.

One other aspect of limberness is that at the catch the horizontal angle of the oar from thwartwise is not at an efficient position to drive the boat, see figure 2. However, at the catch the rower can get his energy started efficiently into the oar for later release, by which time the oar will be at a more efficient position after the first surge, but maybe not at the second surge.

The second surge is likely a combination of the forward "lift" in slicing the blades up through the water in the second half of the doryman's stroke and, possibly, the adverse sudden snapping of the rower's back aft to start the recovery. In effect the rower pulls himself up and aft by yanking on the oars. This sternward momentum of the rower's body is matched by equal forward momentum of the boat at the wrong time. This can be avoided by the rower using a smoother back motion without the yank and/or snapping the back aft. More about this in the next topic, Synchronizing the Rower's To-and-Fro Motion (section 25).

There is a dandy overhead photograph of the wave system of a fast guide boat and the flexing of its oars in WoodenBoat #18. The oars are either the soft maple #13 in Table 1, or their similar birch companions #33 not shown.

It appears that as time passes there may be many more light rowboats, chiefly because they are handled so easily on land and on car tops. If the best performance is to be had from these boats, their oars should probably be very limber. This poses a problem because the very limber woods are not readily available in the high quality of straight grain and freedom from knots that the best limber oars require. The softwoods, even expensive Sitka spruce, lack the limberness needed. Guide-boat oars use soft (red) maple (acer rubrum), birch, and cherry because they exist in the Adirondacks. No truly traditional guide boat uses imported wood species not found in the Adirondacks.

A flexing blade rules out a cupped-spoon shape as it is too rigid. So here a choice for other light boats elsewhere is necessary between a very limber oar with straight blade or the potential improvements possible in a cupped-spoon blade. Maybe the answer is a rigid-spoon blade on a very limber loom extending from grip to neck with reinforcing at the lock.

Although the guide boat and the curragh, along with their oars, are vastly different in appearance and construction, it is fascinating to note the similarity in the uses of their oars and the responses of these boats when lightly loaded. The curraghs were researched over 50 years ago by J. Hornell (see bibliography).

The old curragh designs have existed for centuries largely unchanged in basic form and light construction, except for

the modern planked curraghs. Their speed and seaworthiness are legendary, as well as the resourcefulness, skill, and feats of seamanship of their crews, who didn't hesitate to attack large fish, mammals, and even giant squid. Their recorded history is fascinating reading, and that is only a small part of their history. An ancient craft has stood the test of time because it was good to start with and well adapted to the rough sea conditions of use and limited availability of materials of construction.

{25}

Synchronizing the Rower's To-and-Fro Motion

This tale assumed previously that the rower's to-and-fro motion was neglected in making several other points easier to understand. Let's pick up this loose thread, and weave the rower's motion back and forth through the ancient fabric of fixed-seat rowing. We start with the basic principles and then list some specific synchronizing tips.

The rower's body performs two separate functions. The predominant one is a combination strength and timing function pulling the oars to propel the boat. This is the propelling function.

The other job is a to-and-fro body-weight function, which also involves timing. This is the momentum function, which uses the law of conservation of momentum between the rower and his boat and the resistance laws of a moving boat. Both functions require motion of the rower's body parts, but not necessarily always the same parts concurrently, although that happens luckily at times. This is where the rower's synchronizing skill in blending the two functions becomes the subject of this topic.

The need for getting in sync arises because the surging nature of oar propulsion causes a greater hull resistance through the water than if the same boat was propelled at an equal constant average velocity by a steady thrust of a propeller or sail. And a reduction of surge will result in lower resistance of the boat through the water. So a means of reducing the highest boat velocity at the end of the pull, and increasing the lowest velocity at the end of coasting, should result in less expenditure of rower's energy. It turns out that the rower's body motion to and fro, which is his momentum function, if synchronized, can

reduce the difference between the high and low boat velocities caused by his propelling function. This is done by understanding the law of conservation of momentum, or if one is a natural-born rower, unconsciously using the law without knowing it exists. The law says that the rower by moving his weight <u>within</u> <u>his</u> <u>boat</u>, either to or fro, tends to make the boat go in the opposite direction. His momentum in one direction is balanced by the boat's momentum in the opposite direction. (We assume that for the small momentum velocities for fixed-seat boats, the momentum hull resistance is neglected, but the higher velocity pulling resistance remains).

The momentum of a moving object is defined as its mass times its velocity. For our present purposes we can use mass and weight interchangeably and neglect the gravity constant. If WR and VR are the moving weight and velocity of the rower <u>within</u> his boat in one direction with respect to the combined center of gravity of rower and boat, and WB and VB are the boat's weight and velocity in the opposite direction, also with respect to the same combined C.G., then WRxVR=WBxVB, which can be rewritten VB=VR(WR/WB). So the effective weight ratio of rower to boat is important and varies according to the type of motion, whether sliding or fixed-seat, as well as the net moving weight of rower and boat weight. Here the moving weight of the rower is what he can move <u>within</u> the boat. For fixed-seat rowing he cannot move his legs and butt, which are about half of his total weight and should be included in the boat's weight. Note that the combined C.G. of rower and boat lies on a straight line connecting the rower's and boat's individual C.G.S., and the combined C.G. lies nearer the heavier of the two end C.G.S. in proportion to their weights.

So while the rower using his momentum function is moving forward <u>within</u> the boat, he can by momentum transfer, cause

the boat to tend to move astern. If he does this while pulling the oars using his propelling function, he will reduce the boat's forward velocity through the water to less than it would have been if he hadn't moved forward. Likewise, if he moves aft within the boat, he can increase the boat's forward velocity at a time when the boat is slowing down during coasting. He is having his cake and eating it, by reducing the difference between the high and low surging boat velocities and thereby reducing the hull resistance losses, if he synchronizes his body's momentum function with its propelling function.

Of course, the rower cannot move indefinitely in either direction because he is supposed to stay fixed-seated, but he has time to move a limited amount for the duration of the pull and back again while coasting. Also, the instant he stops moving within the boat, the boat stops its corresponding momentum velocity in the opposite direction.

Since the boat's momentum velocity can be independent of its propelling velocity under the influence of the oars, the two velocities can be superposed on each other. When this is done properly, the rower is in sync and the boat moves easier. Otherwise he is out of sync, and the boat doesn't go as well.

The sliding-seat rower enjoys a much greater momentum effect because practically all of his weight moves through a much greater distance than does that of the fixed-seat rower. In fact, the proper synchronizing of the various body parts is one of the major lessons the sliding-seat rower learns. For us fixed-seaters who have fewer parts to move, there is much to learn by observing both good and bad sliders.

To be sure, it is hard to pull the oars without moving the

body forward, which is a very fortunate circumstance (but not for bow-facing oars, as will be seen later). However, it all depends on how much the oars are moved primarily by the lighter and quicker arms and hands or by the heavier back and shoulders that offers the opportunity for the rower to synchronize his motions.

There is also a kinetic energy function that produces a moderating influence on reducing the high boat velocity on the pull and increasing the low boat velocity when the boat coasts. On the pull, if the rower moves his C.G. forward <u>within</u> the boat it will be going a little faster than the boat, so his body will store a little more K.E. per lb. of his moving weight than the boat. This extra energy must come from the boat's K.E., so the high boat velocity through the water is a little less than it would have been if he hadn't moved forward. This energy effect is like the transfer of momentum effect in moderating the high forward boat velocity. Then during recovery, the rower's C.G. moves aft within the boat and gives up his extra stored energy to the boat to increase its forward velocity, as his momentum velocity does.

Momentum enjoys a peculiar status because it cannot be felt by humans. This discussion about applying momentum to rowing would be briefer if rowers could feel momentum. We can sense a momentum change, which is acceleration, and we can observe the effects of momentum, and reason out its uses in our heads. But momentum itself is elusive, probably because it depends on velocity, which we cannot feel either, except by its change which is acceleration. We only feel acceleration because it requires or produces a force, and we can sense time. There is nothing mysterious about momentum, only that it is intangible. It should be very easy for a rower to get in sync if momentum could be felt.

Let's boil all of the foregoing basics down to the following specific suggestions governing the most effective transfer of momentum between the rower and his boat. The general rule is to use the arms mostly at the ends of both pulling and recovery strokes and the heavier back in the middle of both strokes. And the arm and back motions should blend into each other in a way to synchronize the momentum function with the propelling function. The same applies to K.E.

1. Beginning of Pull. Move the rower's heavier back toward the bow only after the lighter arms and hands have secured a quick and firm catch as explained previously in Grab at the Catch (section 21); otherwise the premature forward motion of the heavier body will tend to kick the boat astern when the boat is at or near its lowest forward velocity.

2. During the Pull. Move the heavier body parts forward fastest when the forward component of pull on the oars is greatest. For the horizontal sweeping stroke, this is generally near thwartwise oar position where the position efficiency is greatest (see figure 2). For the doryman's stroke and the first peak on curve F, figure 14, start the back toward the bow during the surging descent of the blade through the water, but not before in order to soften the surge. Use only part of the available back motion and reserve the rest for the balance of the pull, including the second surge. Keep a continuation of the body and arms moving forward during the whole pull to reduce the high boat velocity due to the pull of the oars, using the arms mainly at stroke ends.

3. <u>End of Pull</u>. A crítical time is just before the end of the pull when some rowers (even gifted ones, and most of us on occasion) anticipate the recovery too soon and give the oars a final yank to help reverse their body motion toward the stern. The error is in accelerating the boat forward with both the yank for more power, and the sudden simultaneous movement of their back aft when the boat is already moving forward its fastest. This is not using the back's momentum to moderate the high forward boat velocity as should be done. This just increases the fuss and lost energy in the water at the bow, and bobs the bow down with even more fuss. Movies of races in light boats clearly show this common error, especially in slow-motion projection. Furthermore, the end of the pull is an inefficient position to apply a burst of energy (see figure 2), unless the after stroke is very short. The rower should be easing his pull using mostly his arms before lifting the blades out of water with the minimum of splashing turbulence in the puddles.

   The second surge of the doryman's stroke, when the blade is rising through the water, should not be delayed as long as showed by the right-hand peak of figure 14, Curve F. This peak shows the same disadvantages of the end-of-pull yank on the oar where the boat velocity is near its maximum. It would be more efficient to start the blade up sooner and with a longer ascent time to smooth out the surge. Also, this last doryman's surge could be softened with the last bit of back motion toward the bow.

4. <u>Beginning of Recovery</u>. The boat is going forward

fastest then, so avoid as much back motion aft as possible with its accompanying added forward-momentum velocity of the boat. Don't snap the back aft then with the oars out of water. Start the recovery stroke mostly with the lighter arms. There should be no hesitation of the oars at either end of both strokes. That is just wasting time when the boat velocity is decaying.

5. <u>During Recovery</u>. Use a combination of arm and back motion aft during the whole recovery stroke, with the arms mainly at stroke ends to give a smooth reversal of the oars. Move the back aft fastest mostly for the middle of the stroke and in the after quadrant when the forward boat velocity is decaying and a forward boat momentum velocity assist would be most helpful.

6. <u>End of Recovery</u>. Use mostly arm action near and at the end of the recovery stroke to provide a smooth and quick reverse of the oars without back action.

7. Synchronizing the rower's arm and back momentum motions with the pull of the oars also applies when there is more than one rower aboard. Collectively, they will do better if they are all in practiced sync.

8. Some light rowboats susceptible to surging, such as the guide boat, have a rower forward and a paddler aft. They might be racing or just cruising. The paddler should pull a long paddle with as big a blade as he can swing deep in the water to match the rower's stroke rate and move his body forward on the pull in sync with the rower.

9. Some rowers, depending on conditions, will use a shorter stroke at higher rate, keeping the oars near thwartwise for higher efficiency, per figure 2. Obviously, the higher the rate, the nearer oar propulsion approaches steady thrust, and the less the need to get in sync. In this situation the rower will use less back motion, because he can move his arms faster. Actually, it is just as well for some of us codgers with stiff backs in our later years.

10. A heavy rower has a disadvantage, unless endowed with compensating strength, of causing more hull displacement and resistance. However, greater weight also can help by producing more rower's momentum, especially if it is more concentrated in his upper body, which moves to and fro the most for the fixed-seated rower. But he has to move his greater weight skillfully in sync.

Bow-Facing Oars. If the reader has rowed a light boat with bow-facing oars, reelfoot lake style, or equivalent, such as those brought to Mystic's annual June small craft workshop by Mr. Myron Young, he will have had a very novel, fascinating, and instructive experience if he has only rowed facing aft for years. Everything is reversed, including the conditioned steering reflexes, and the momentum transfer between rower and boat.

The first time out, the rower suddenly finds himself in a pickle and has to slowly learn again to row differently. His to-and-fro motion is 180 degrees out of sync. When he pulls the oars to make the boat go forward, his back is moving astern, which by conservation of momentum is additionally moving the boat ahead and tending to

unexpectedly snatch the boat out from under himself at the highest forward boat velocity. This is just the opposite of what he should do with his back motion to slow the boat's maximum forward velocity when he rows facing aft.

Likewise, for the recovery he pulls his body forward by his stomach muscles, which complain. And in moving his body forward it tends to send the boat astern to slow the boat even further when the boat is already approaching its minimum forward velocity.

The net effect of his body motion to and fro is much greater disparity between the high forward boat velocity on the pull and the lower forward velocity on the recovery stroke. And with increased hull resistance losses, the average boat speed drops. His momentum transfer is out of sync. This shows by adverse comparison how important in normal rowing in a surging boat it is to get the to-and-fro body in sync. However, the bow-facing oars let the rower see where he is going on a crowded watercourse, or a stump-covered reelfoot lake. In using these oars in a light boat, the rower should move his body to and fro as little as possible and depend on his arms. If the boat is heavy, it won't surge much so the rower doesn't have to be particular how he rows in ordinary usage.

Here is a list of desirable oar characteristics that increase the responsiveness of oars and help get the rower in sync. See Table 1 for some of them. They enhance the transfer of momentum between rower and boat because timing is more precise.

1. Light weight and some spring;

2. Near perfect balance to suit a particular rower;

3. Low inertia force, F, at the grips, both horizontally and vertically, to facilitate fast blade action, particularly at the catch;

4. Long inner loom length to allow rower a long reach and plenty of body movement. This also promotes greater transfer of kinetic energy between rower and boat and greater impulse;

5. Some blade dig angle at the catch to start a fast grab so the rower's body motion can start as soon as possible;

6. Low blade buoyancy to help a fast grab;

7. Pick an oar with a low enough pull number Y, when going up wind to allow a high enough stroke rate to more nearly approach steady thrust to counteract the boat's slowing down on the recovery; also use plenty of back motion to reduce the surge by momentum transfer;

8. In going down wind, pick an oar with a higher pull number so the stroke rate won't be too fast to wear out the rower. And besides, the wind resistance is an aid, not a hindrance to the boat's progress. So it doesn't slow down as much on the recovery;

9. Large enough hand grips to avoid blisters. It is hard to get into sync if uncomfortable;

10. Smooth running and quiet oarlocks that give better control of blade action and smoother timing;

11. Oarlocks that give repeatable and dependable blade

dig angle to enhance precision timing;

12. While not an oar characteristic, the stretcher must be far enough aft of the locks so the rowers legs will be almost straight, and the knees low enough, to allow the rower to bend aft as far as he can without interference. Being supple helps.

For us fixed-seaters in the lighter boats, getting in sync is most necessary to attain that delightful feeling of being "in the groove," that at times seems to let us almost effortlessly rattle off the miles in a nice day's row.

Lastly, figure 18 is a chain graph of momentum, which makes it very easy to determine how far the boat will go in one direction when the rower moves in the opposite direction. Just as the rower is confined to a particular range of to-and-fro motion within the boat, the boat is also restricted by the interchange of momentum between it and the rower on how far it can move in the opposite direction. To use the graph all we need are the weights of the rower and boat and how far the estimated C.G. of the rower's upper body moves to and fro in his boat. The fixed-seat math automatically detaches the rower's legs and butt from his total weight, and attaches them back on the boat's weight at the right spot. So we don't have to think about that.

Note that the distance the boat moves through the water is proportional to the distance the rower's C.G. moves. If the rower doesn't move his C.G. much, just rowing with his arms, the boat won't move to and fro much either. And, of course, the boat won't start and stop it's momentum motion until the rower starts and stops his motion. So the rower has a convenient momentum throttle by how much he moves his back and when. But he cannot feel the momentum he is

throttling.

There should be no restrictions on the rower's range of action, such as high knees and legs, bulky clothing, inner looms of the oars too short, or the locks too close or too far from the rower. Being able to stand up straight and bend over to touch the floor with one's fingers, and the knees straight, is good for rowing.

Figure 19 shows the mathematical derivation for figure 18, and is included for those who might wonder how the graph was made. The graph shows how greater range of boat motion is had when the rower's weight is increased, the boat's weight is decreased, and the rower's to-and-fro motion is increased.

{26}
Rowing Heavy vs. Light Boats

Sometimes at a small boat gathering a spontaneous discussion will erupt on the rowing merits of heavier versus lighter boats in going to windward against a breezy chop. The opposing sides are usually set in their thoughts, and no agreement is ever reached. Doubtless, the following comments won't alter anybody's views, but I hope they will cast light on how heavy and light boats respond to oars, how oars can be used to compensate for a boat's weight, and how the wind and water conditions affect the design of a rowboat. Sooner or later we find ourselves in a variety of boats, if we are really interested in all rowboats.

Many of us own light boats out of necessity, if we don't live on the water and must handle them on land or on car-top. Also the Adirondack guide boat and all its equipment had to be light for the carry from one watercourse to the next. Some of the light boats, particularly the guide boat among the traditional types, also make superb racing boats, because they are so responsive to the oars.

Suppose we start in a quiet cove with a flotilla of different row boat types, each with a single rower weighing about 165 lbs., and proceed shortly out to open water, first against a breeze and then against white caps and maybe Neptune's horses. By starting out in a calm cove we might agree at the beginning on a few things, even though later we might not.

Calm Water. First, the most striking feature of a rowboat is its surging progress, with the surge rate set by the stroke rate. This feature is lacking in sail- and powerboats. A heavy rowboat will surge, but not very much.

The lighter the boat, usually the more pronounced is its surge. If we include a racing single shell, weighing only 30 lbs. or so, in our flotilla, the surge is very evident. Sometimes, depending on the rower's skill, the shell almost seems to come to a stop, and be accelerated each stroke from a standing start. However, a good rower can do better than that. As we proceed up the scale of weights of boats in the flotilla to the guide boats, Rushton's rowboats, several small but different Rangeleys, St. Lawrence skiffs, Whitehalls, peapods, dorys, and the heavier loaded work boats, the degree of surge becomes less and the average speed is less. Note that all of these latter boats are fixed-seat craft as originally intended in these articles.

I doubt that Isaac Newton ever rowed a light racing single shell, but he must have been pretty certain that his second law of motion, F=mxa, would apply to anything that came rowing into sight. Here the terms are defined the same as in <u>Rowboat Surging</u> (section 23) so they won't be repeated here.

There is one other force on the boat in the calm cove, and that is the hull resistance in the water, RW, which retards it. Note that RW isn't constant, but is very speed dependent. In fact, none of the terms we meet here are constant, except g, and we will assume W is also, in a fixed location for each boat.

Then a=gx(FT-RW)/W, where FT-RW is the net force forward on the boat, and we are ready for some general qualitative observations. This expression tells us that at any instant, the stronger the push of the water forward against the oar blades during a stroke, the greater the acceleration, a, will be. The more the resistance of the boat through the water, since it has a negative sign, the less a will be. And the lighter the weight of boat and rower, W, since it

is in the denominator, the greater a will be. So the racing single shell is a good example. The FT is high for a trained athlete; the water resistance, RW, is very low because the shell produces almost no wave resistance, its wetted surface and skin friction are low, and the hull is nicely streamlined so its eddy resistance is low; and W is about as low as a rowboat could be. All of these factors make for high acceleration on the pull.

When the oars are out of the water, FT becomes zero. So with only RW affecting the shell's motion, it must decelerate (because a is then negative), and the shell will do so fast, because W is small. Since we are dealing with rowboat motion after the boat has left shore and reached a more or less uniform average speed, naturally, there won't be acceleration on the pull unless there is deceleration on the recovery.

Actually, the fore-and-aft motion of the rower's body with respect to the boat, has an effect on the boat's speed. This effect can be maximized, see Synchronizing the Rower's To-and-Fro Motion (section 25). For the sake of clarity here, the to-and-fro body motion is neglected.

When Newton's law is applied to a heavy working rowboat where the rower has other things to do beside setting a speed record, his oar force, FT, is much lower, and the weight, W, is much greater. So the acceleration, a, is much less and almost imperceptible, although it's still there. Consequently his deceleration is also low, so the surging effect is less pronounced. If the heavy boat has easy lines, such as an old 20- to 23-ft. St. Lawrence skiff, so the water resistance, RW, is low, then the deceleration is very low, and the boat has a lot of "carry" and can be rowed with a slow stroke, because it doesn't slow down much between pulls. Therefore it doesn't have to be accelerated

much on the pull. However, in the cove, the heavy boat will never catch up to the light boat, if it also has good form with a lower water resistance and the two rowers are more or less matched in strength and skill, because the lighter-displacement boat has less wave resistance and less wetted surface and skin friction.

There is one thing about the lighter boat in the cove: the rower can't wait too long between pulls if his boat decelerates too fast. Otherwise its almost like getting the boat started from scratch at each stroke. So he must row with a faster stroke. And the light guide boat should have very limber oars as mentioned in <u>Limber Oars</u> (section 24).

Before we leave the cove, it is very instructive for the rowers to change boats to see what the other fellow has to work with. But let's keep the oars with the rowers. When the light boat's rower gets into the heavy boat, he is immediately struck by the harder pull his own oars now have. They feel like something has firmly grabbed him. In fact, it is the lower acceleration of the heavy boat that upsets his pull expectation and timing. The boat lacks the fast pick-up feel of his light boat, which has higher acceleration. So he'll have to get used to a different feel of the pull, and it will be a longer pull (time-wise). There is more impulse per stroke with a slower stroke. The catch will be different too. If he just calms down and doesn't fight his oars, the boat may do alright. It's average speed will be OK for that type of boat. But it takes longer to get the heavy boat up to speed. It's the difference between driving a flivver and a Mack truck. Likewise, the heavy boat rower, when he gets into the light boat, thinks he is riding a jack rabbit and has to modify his style with a faster but easier stroke.

<u>Against Wind</u>. Let's move out of the cove into breezy, but

fairly smooth, open water. The racing shell will take one look and say, "Uh-uh." For one thing, his stability depends on his oars balancing his craft in calm water, so we'll leave him behind. But, there is a sturdy Eskimo with us in his very light hunting kayak or a modern man in his modern sea kayak to take the single shell's place. True, the kayak is paddled, not rowed. But Sir Isaac is a friend of all who propel a boat by an intermittent motion. Let's take the breeze against us at first, and simply subtract a wind resistance term, RB, from the net force in the numerator. So Isaac looks like: a=gx(FT-RW-RB)/W. And here, in addition to light and heavy boats, there are boats with more or less windage, RB, of the hull, rower, oars, paddle, etc.

Windage will slow all boats because it reduces their acceleration on the pull, and increases their deceleration between pulls when FT=0. So now, if we compare a light and heavy boat, each with the same windage, we might have to row both boats at a faster stroke than we did in the cove, but more so the lighter boat to keep it from slowing too much between pulls. But still, the lighter boat with its lower hull resistance, RW, should be easier to row at the same comparable speed as the heavy boat. So the faster stroke of the lighter boat needn't take more rower's energy than the slower stroke of the heavy boat. Naturally, for the faster stroke, tuned oars can be moved easier.

Another advantage of maintaining a faster stroke in the lighter boat is that the propulsion efficiency of the oars, particularly at the catch, is always greater when the boat speed is kept up. It's sort of a boot-strap effect (see Oar Efficiency (section 14)). The Eskimo with a double-bladed paddle can have a much faster stroke than a rower. This is a great help against the breeze. The wind resistance, RB, of the kayak is very low, which conserves

energy, and by Sir Isaac, reduces the deceleration between pulls. This is the way to go in a lot of wind, low freeboard with spray covers if necessary in a rowboat.

So several things are really needed to make a light boat go against the wind. The oars should be tuned and used with a high enough stroke rate, and they should be short enough from the lock out to the blade center of pressure to get the faster stroke without an excessively hard pull, when the boat is running slower through the water (see Slip (section 6)). This is the condition for which I carry along shorter oars. And the boat should be designed with low wind resistance for windward work. Here it is noted that simply taking the same lines of a traditionally heavier boat and building it much lighter will raise the freeboard and wind resistance. So some thought should be given to decreasing wind resistance when a boat is built much lighter than its ancestor.

Against Chop. Now let's move the flotilla out into more open water against a chop. Meeting waves head-on will add a chop resistance, RC, to the net force on the boat. So Sir Isaac's expression will now look like: a=gx(FT-RW-RB-RC)/W; where the chop is an intermittent thrust against the boat and it can decrease acceleration on the pull, and increase deceleration between pulls. Here again a little higher stroke rate will help a light boat keep going and maintain higher propulsion efficiency. Sharp lines forward, both water lines and steep sections, will help either a heavy or light boat manage a chop with less fuss in the water at the bow, and so less lost energy from the rower.

Pounding a rowboat to windward absorbs the rower's energy in thrown spray. My 18-ft. rowboat, weighing only 75 lbs., can be driven fast enough to pound in rough water in spite of very sharp lines if the waves are steep enough and come

at the right interval. The boat will shoot off one crest and drop into the next. This can happen in a breezy tide rip, and it tells me the boat is going too fast for the conditions. So I just slow down a bit with an easier, but not slower, stroke. So there are ways to get a light boat with low resistances to windward in rough water by using the right size of tuned limber oars with a faster stroke.

Adding Ballast. Some folks like to add ballast when going upwind. (Be sure the boat won't sink, if it fills by accident). In this case a=gx(FT-RW-RB-RC)/(W+). Here both acceleration on the pull and deceleration between pulls are decreased by the added weight. Since the added displacement should increase hull resistance, RW, through the water, there is some speed reduction. To the extent that the extra weight has decreased freeboard, there will be a slight decrease in wind resistance, RB.

The most effective way to add weight going upwind is with another rower doing useful work. The total weight is not doubled, because the boat's weight isn't doubled. Then: a=gx(2FT-(RW+)-RB-RC)/(W+). The extra weight increases the water resistance. The wind resistance may not change much because less freeboard offsets the windage of the second rower and his oars. Here it is very likely that the acceleration on the pull is increased due to the greater force and the deceleration between pulls is decreased because of the greater weight. So the boat travels faster and the oar efficiency is higher. The water resistance increases, but not enough to slow the boat down overall. So adding another rower is the best way to go upwind. Not necessarily because Newton said so, but rather because he laid his finger on the principles that say so.

Adding ballast to trim a rowboat for various reasons, such as balancing a passenger, or altering the underwater

lateral plane or freeboard wind resistance to make a boat track better, or keep a bow down so it doesn't scatter as much water in a chop, is a separate subject related to the tuning of a rowboat rather than the use of oars. However, to the extent such ballast additions make a rowboat go better, there will be increased propulsion efficiency of the oars.

Downwind. Now it is time to turn the flotilla around to take the wind and chop with us back to the cove. Nobody complains much whether they are in a light or heavy boat. The pull on the oars will be less as the boats go faster and the lighter boats can row a slower rate than upwind. Some of the light boats could change over to longer oars for a sleigh ride (see Slip (section 6)) so they can keep F and impulse up. The water resistance, RW, will be increased some because the boat moves faster. The wind and chop resistances, RB and RC, are now reversed so Sir Isaac becomes: a=gx(FT-RW+RB+RC)/W. Then on the pull, the acceleration is greater than when going up wind. And between pulls, when FT=0, the deceleration is less. Consequently, the average boat speed is greater than when going upwind. If we stop rowing downwind long enough, and coast, then a practically steady drifting speed is reached where FT=0, and RW=RB+RC. Then there are no acceleration or deceleration surges when a=0, except for a little surging from the waves going our way.

So Isaac Newton has provided a very simple and fundamental way to correlate our thinking in a consistent manner on the various situations we meet rowing different boats, how to use oars, and why light boats should be designed for the least resistances.

Note that prams and similar acting rowboats are omitted here because their high resistance characteristics of

water, wind, and chop, don't allow them to get very far compared to other boats under rough conditions. Light boats must be easily driven for the human engine has very small power.

A Last Word

While it may seem that undue attention has been paid to racing in this discussion of "Pleasure Oars," the racing folks, their boats, and their oars deserve close scrutiny because much can be learned to advance the design and use of our pleasure oars in fixed-seat boats. Innovations are more likely to spring up first among racers because theirs is a very strong incentive. (In the Adirondacks, they sometimes race for money, like in the olden days). Their physical condition is usually pretty good, and the first one home often has used his wits, skill, energy, and equipment more effectively than some stronger or younger rowers behind him, all characteristics that can enhance our enjoyment in non-competitive rowing under all sorts of conditions, even though we do not intend to race.

Rowing, far from being "dog work," can be an exhilarating challenge in the right setting, river rowing in particular with its winds and currents. The big St. Lawrence and the Maine tidal reversing rivers are tops on a cool bright October day. On the Maine coast, it is a handy day's row from Christmas Cove up to Damariscotta for hot fish chowder and blueberry muffins, before returning, often against a strong challenging wind, when an ebb current is useless, except through the "fast waters." Having good boats and oars can lead to some fabulous experiences year after year with marvelous memories. I wish that 60 years ago I knew what I know now. So I hope that some young people will read this and enhance a lifetime of enjoyment in rowing versatile fixed-seat boats. I have rowed many different kinds of boats, ranging from the fastest sliding-seat singles to the heavy Norwegian fishing boats, and still find a good, light fixed-seater the most fun and adaptable to all around use. But it has to be a good one, well tuned, and with tuned oars.

Appendix

	Subject	Reference Section	
Table 1	Oar Characteristics	{3}	Balance
Figures 1a-h	Slip Diagrams	{6}	Slip
Figure 2	Position Efficiency	{10}	Stroke Rate
Figure 3	Force Lever	{11}	Leverage
Figure 4	Oar Efficiency	{14}	Oar Efficiency
Figure 5	Spoon Oar, Mid-stroke	{14}	Oar Efficiency
Figure 6	Base Oar Efficiency	{14}	Oar Efficiency
Figure 7	Base Oar Efficiency	{14}	Oar Efficiency
Figure 8	Dig Angle	{15}	Blade Area & Shape
Figure 9	Doryman's Stroke	{15}	Blade Area & Shape
Figure 10	Oar Selection Calc's	{16}	Selection of Oars
Figure 11	Oar Rating Chart	{16}	Selection of Oars
Figure 12	Oar Selection Chart	{16}	Selection of Oars
Figure 13	Straight Blade Shapes	{16}	Selection of Oars
Figure 14	Impulse Diagram	{20}	Impulse
Figure 15	Derivation of True Dig Angle	{22}	Blade Dig Angle
Figure 16	Graph of True Dig Angle	{22}	Blade Dig Angle
Figure 17	Irish Curragh Oars	{23}	Rowboat Surging
Figure 18	Synchronizing Graph	{25}	Synchronizing
Figure 19	Synchronizing Derivation	{25}	Synchronizing

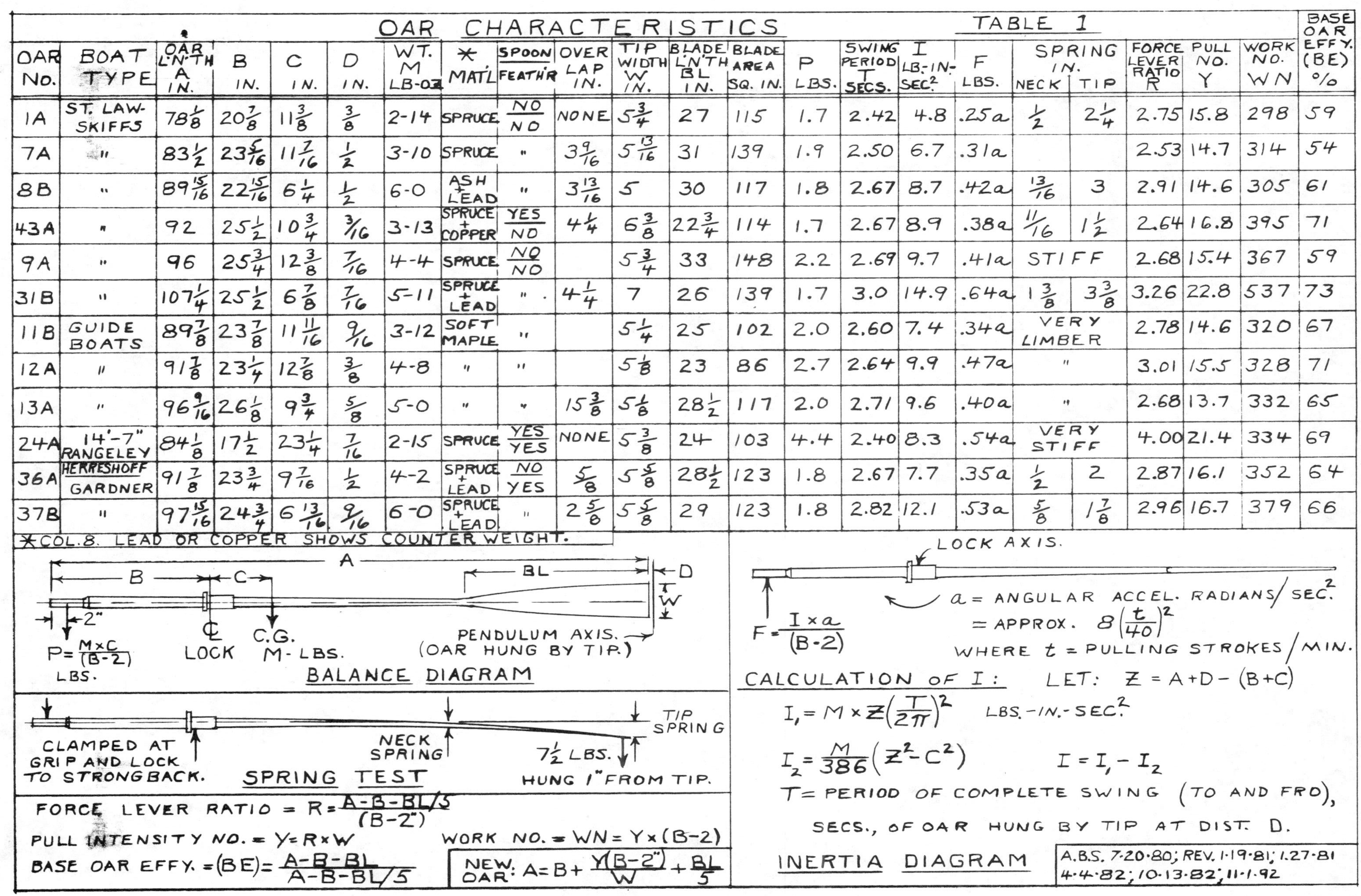

OAR CHARACTERISTICS

TABLE 1

OAR No.	BOAT TYPE	OAR L'N'TH A IN.	B IN.	C IN.	D IN.	WT. M LB-OZ	* MAT'L	SPOON / FEATH'R	OVER LAP IN.	TIP WIDTH W IN.	BLADE L'N'TH BL IN.	BLADE AREA SQ. IN.	P LBS.	SWING PERIOD T SECS.	I LB.-IN.-SEC.^{2}	F LBS.	SPRING IN. NECK	SPRING IN. TIP	FORCE LEVER RATIO R	PULL NO. Y	WORK NO. WN	BASE OAR EFFY. (BE) %
1A	ST. LAW. SKIFFS	$78\frac{1}{8}$	$20\frac{7}{8}$	$11\frac{3}{8}$	$\frac{3}{8}$	2-14	SPRUCE	NO / NO	NONE	$5\frac{3}{4}$	27	115	1.7	2.42	4.8	.25a	$\frac{1}{2}$	$2\frac{1}{4}$	2.75	15.8	298	59
7A	"	$83\frac{1}{2}$	$23\frac{5}{16}$	$11\frac{7}{16}$	$\frac{1}{2}$	3-10	SPRUCE	"	$3\frac{9}{16}$	$5\frac{13}{16}$	31	139	1.9	2.50	6.7	.31a			2.53	14.7	314	54
8B	"	$89\frac{15}{16}$	$22\frac{15}{16}$	$6\frac{1}{4}$	$\frac{1}{2}$	6-0	ASH + LEAD	"	$3\frac{13}{16}$	5	30	117	1.8	2.67	8.7	.42a	$\frac{13}{16}$	3	2.91	14.6	305	61
43A	"	92	$25\frac{1}{2}$	$10\frac{3}{4}$	$\frac{3}{16}$	3-13	SPRUCE + COPPER	YES / NO	$4\frac{1}{4}$	$6\frac{3}{8}$	$22\frac{3}{4}$	114	1.7	2.67	8.9	.38a	$\frac{11}{16}$	$1\frac{1}{2}$	2.64	16.8	395	71
9A	"	96	$25\frac{3}{4}$	$12\frac{3}{8}$	$\frac{7}{16}$	4-4	SPRUCE	NO / NO		$5\frac{3}{4}$	33	148	2.2	2.69	9.7	.41a	STIFF		2.68	15.4	367	59
31B	"	$107\frac{1}{4}$	$25\frac{1}{2}$	$6\frac{7}{8}$	$\frac{7}{16}$	5-11	SPRUCE + LEAD	"	$4\frac{1}{4}$	7	26	139	1.7	3.0	14.9	.64a	$1\frac{3}{8}$	$3\frac{3}{8}$	3.26	22.8	537	73
11B	GUIDE BOATS	$89\frac{7}{8}$	$23\frac{7}{8}$	$11\frac{11}{16}$	$\frac{9}{16}$	3-12	SOFT MAPLE	"		$5\frac{1}{4}$	25	102	2.0	2.60	7.4	.34a	VERY LIMBER		2.78	14.6	320	67
12A	"	$91\frac{1}{8}$	$23\frac{1}{4}$	$12\frac{7}{8}$	$\frac{3}{8}$	4-8	"	"		$5\frac{1}{8}$	23	86	2.7	2.64	9.9	.47a	"		3.01	15.5	328	71
13A	"	$96\frac{9}{16}$	$26\frac{1}{8}$	$9\frac{3}{4}$	$\frac{5}{8}$	5-0	"	"	$15\frac{3}{8}$	$5\frac{1}{8}$	$28\frac{1}{2}$	117	2.0	2.71	9.6	.40a	"		2.68	13.7	332	65
24A	14'-7" RANGELEY	$84\frac{1}{8}$	$17\frac{1}{2}$	$23\frac{1}{4}$	$\frac{7}{16}$	2-15	SPRUCE	YES / YES	NONE	$5\frac{3}{8}$	24	103	4.4	2.40	8.3	.54a	VERY STIFF		4.00	21.4	334	69
36A	HERRESHOFF GARDNER	$91\frac{7}{8}$	$23\frac{3}{4}$	$9\frac{7}{16}$	$\frac{1}{2}$	4-2	SPRUCE + LEAD	NO / YES	$\frac{5}{8}$	$5\frac{5}{8}$	$28\frac{1}{2}$	123	1.8	2.67	7.7	.35a	$\frac{1}{2}$	2	2.87	16.1	352	64
37B	"	$97\frac{15}{16}$	$24\frac{3}{4}$	$6\frac{13}{16}$	$\frac{9}{16}$	6-0	SPRUCE + LEAD	"	$2\frac{5}{8}$	$5\frac{5}{8}$	29	123	1.8	2.82	12.1	.53a	$\frac{5}{8}$	$1\frac{7}{8}$	2.96	16.7	379	66

* COL. 8. LEAD OR COPPER SHOWS COUNTER WEIGHT.

BALANCE DIAGRAM

SPRING TEST

FORCE LEVER RATIO = $R=\frac{A-B-BL/5}{(B-2")}$

PULL INTENSITY NO. = $Y=R\times W$

WORK NO. = $WN = Y\times(B-2)$

BASE OAR EFFY. = (BE) = $\frac{A-B-BL}{A-B-BL/5}$

NEW OAR: $A=B+\frac{Y(B-2")}{W}+\frac{BL}{5}$

$F=\frac{I\times a}{(B-2)}$

a = ANGULAR ACCEL. RADIANS/SEC.^{2} = APPROX. $8\left(\frac{t}{40}\right)^2$ WHERE t = PULLING STROKES/MIN.

CALCULATION OF I: LET: $Z = A+D-(B+C)$

$I_1 = M\times Z\left(\frac{T}{2\pi}\right)^2$ LBS.-IN.-SEC.^{2}

$I_2=\frac{M}{386}\left(Z^2-C^2\right)$ $\quad I = I_1 - I_2$

T = PERIOD OF COMPLETE SWING (TO AND FRO), SECS., OF OAR HUNG BY TIP AT DIST. D.

INERTIA DIAGRAM

A.B.S. 7·20·80; REV. 1·19·81; 1·27·81 4·4·82; 10·13·82; 11·1·92

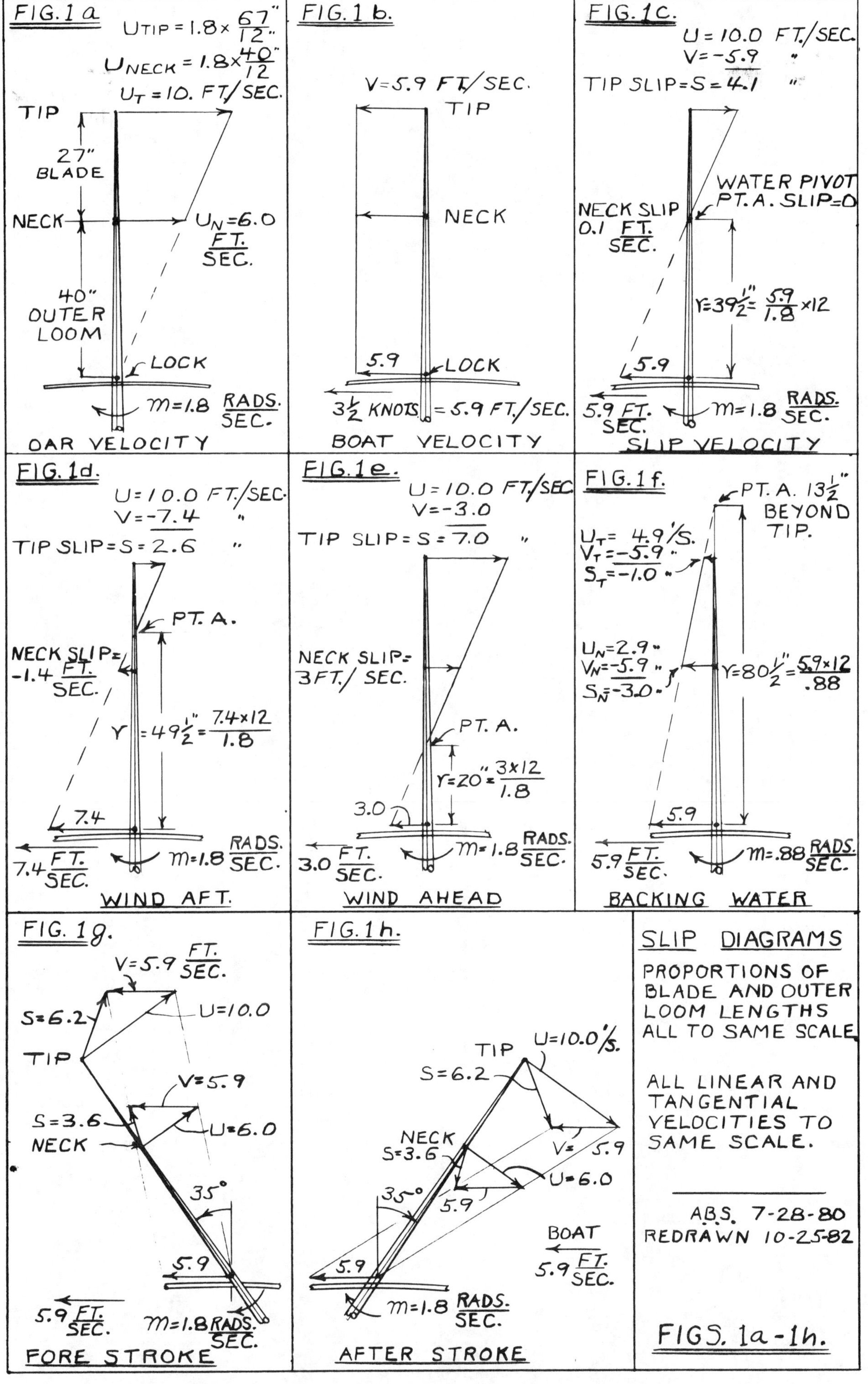
FIG. 1 a
UTIP = 1.8 × 67"/12"
UNECK = 1.8 × 40"/12
UT = 10. FT./SEC.
TIP
27" BLADE
NECK
UN = 6.0 FT./SEC.
40" OUTER LOOM
LOCK
m = 1.8 RADS./SEC.
OAR VELOCITY
FIG. 1 b.
V = 5.9 FT./SEC.
TIP
NECK
5.9
LOCK
3½ KNOTS = 5.9 FT./SEC.
BOAT VELOCITY
FIG. 1 c.
U = 10.0 FT./SEC.
V = -5.9 "
TIP SLIP = S = 4.1 "
WATER PIVOT PT. A. SLIP = O
NECK SLIP 0.1 FT./SEC.
Y = 39½" = 5.9/1.8 × 12
5.9
5.9 FT./SEC.
m = 1.8 RADS./SEC.
SLIP VELOCITY
FIG. 1 d.
U = 10.0 FT./SEC.
V = -7.4 "
TIP SLIP = S = 2.6 "
PT. A.
NECK SLIP = -1.4 FT./SEC.
Y = 49½" = 7.4×12/1.8
7.4
7.4 FT./SEC.
m = 1.8 RADS./SEC.
WIND AFT.
FIG. 1 e.
U = 10.0 FT./SEC.
V = -3.0
TIP SLIP = S = 7.0 "
NECK SLIP = 3 FT./SEC.
PT. A.
Y = 20" = 3×12/1.8
3.0
3.0 FT./SEC.
m = 1.8 RADS./SEC.
WIND AHEAD
FIG. 1 f.
PT. A. 13½" BEYOND TIP.
UT = 4.9'/S.
VT = -5.9 "
ST = -1.0 "
UN = 2.9 "
VN = -5.9 "
SN = -3.0 "
Y = 80½" = 5.9×12/.88
5.9
5.9 FT./SEC.
m = .88 RADS./SEC.
BACKING WATER
FIG. 1 g.
V = 5.9 FT./SEC.
S = 6.2
U = 10.0
TIP
V = 5.9
S = 3.6
U = 6.0
NECK
35°
5.9
5.9 FT./SEC.
m = 1.8 RADS./SEC.
FORE STROKE
FIG. 1 h.
TIP
U = 10.0'/S.
S = 6.2
NECK
S = 3.6
V = 5.9
U = 6.0
35°
5.9
5.9
BOAT
5.9 FT./SEC.
m = 1.8 RADS./SEC.
AFTER STROKE
SLIP DIAGRAMS
PROPORTIONS OF BLADE AND OUTER LOOM LENGTHS ALL TO SAME SCALE.
ALL LINEAR AND TANGENTIAL VELOCITIES TO SAME SCALE.
ABS. 7-28-80
REDRAWN 10-25-82
FIGS. 1a - 1h.

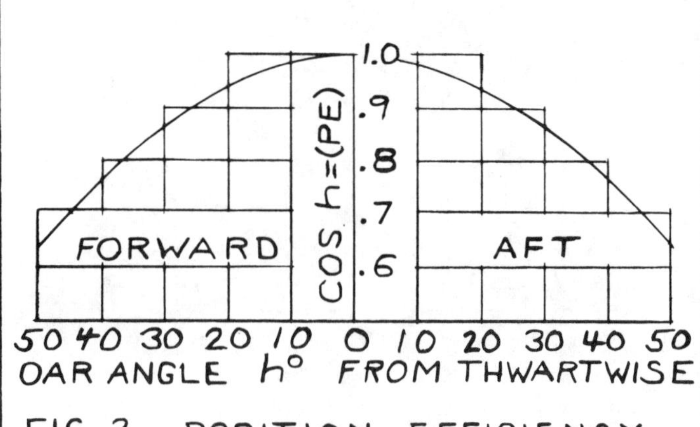

FIG. 2. POSITION EFFICIENCY

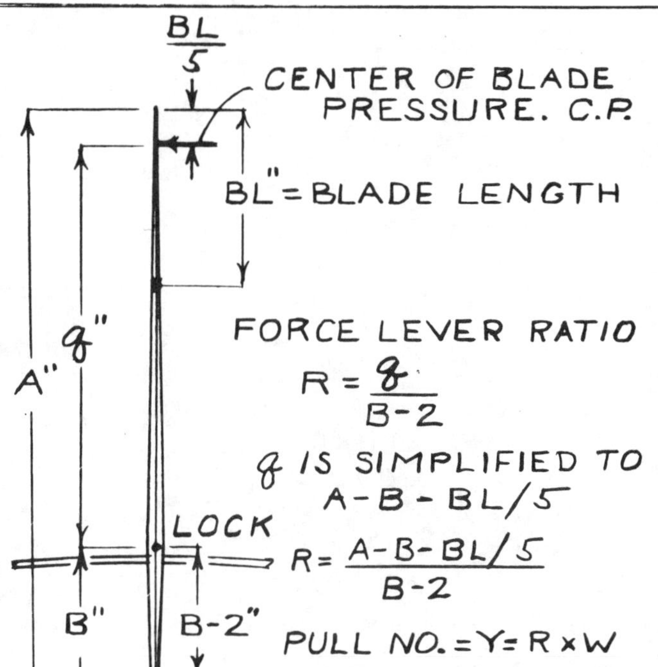

FIG. 3. FORCE LEVER

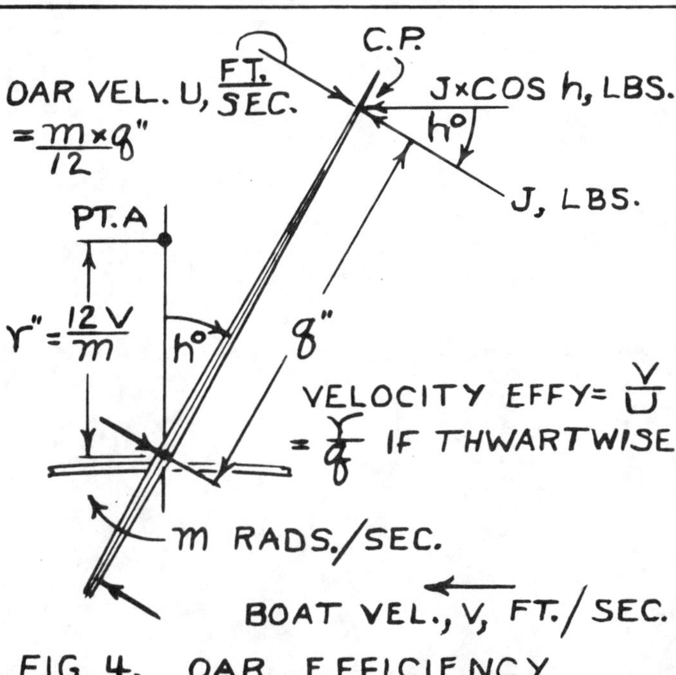

FIG. 4. OAR EFFICIENCY

SHOWS ADDED HYDRODYNAMIC THRUST FORWARD WHEN BLADE MOVES DEEPLY DOWN AND UP. FLAT AFT FACE AND CROWNED BOW FACE. NO RIDGES.

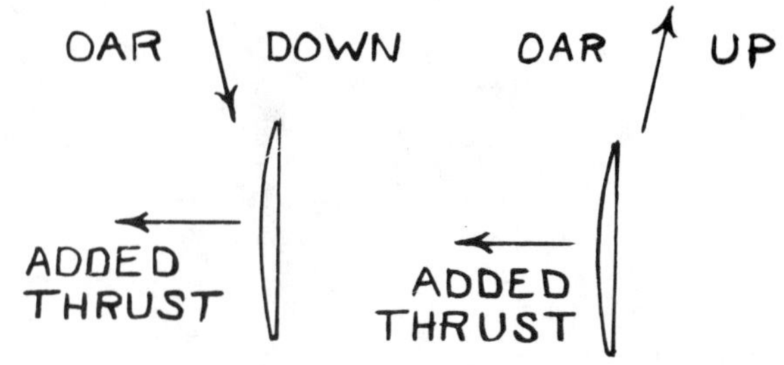

FIG. 9. DORYMAN'S STROKE

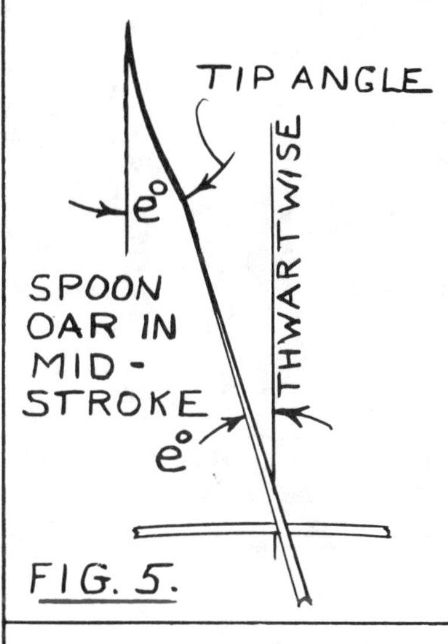

FIG. 5.

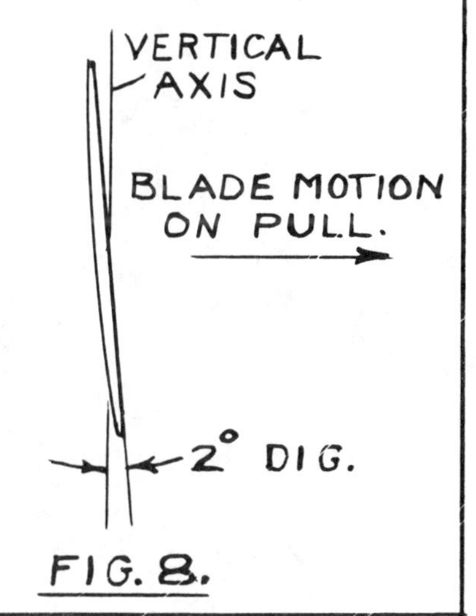

FIG. 8.

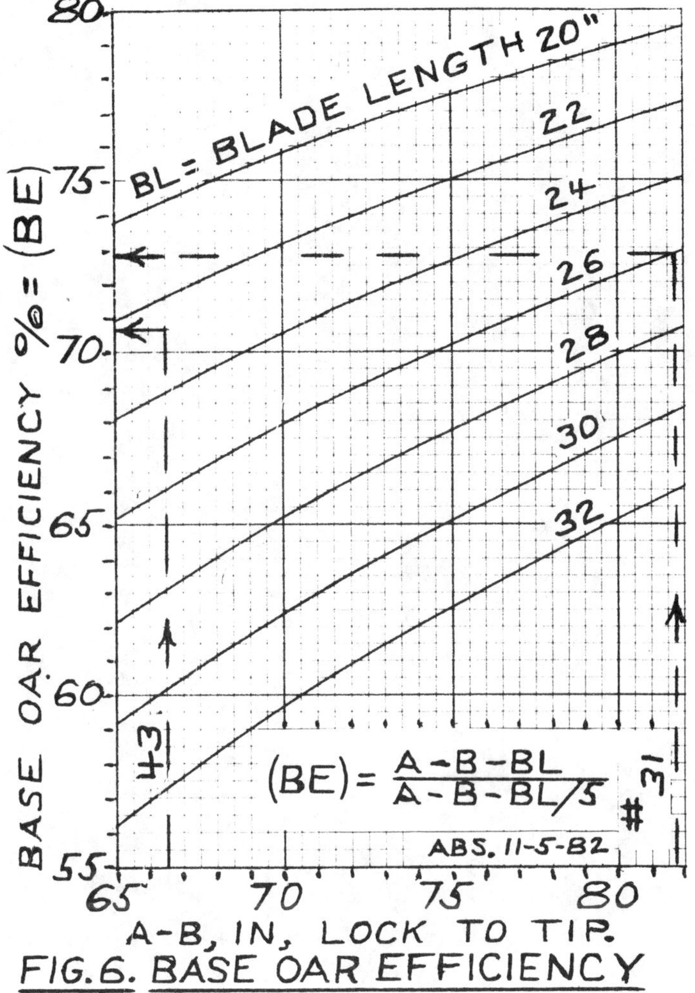

FIG. 6. BASE OAR EFFICIENCY

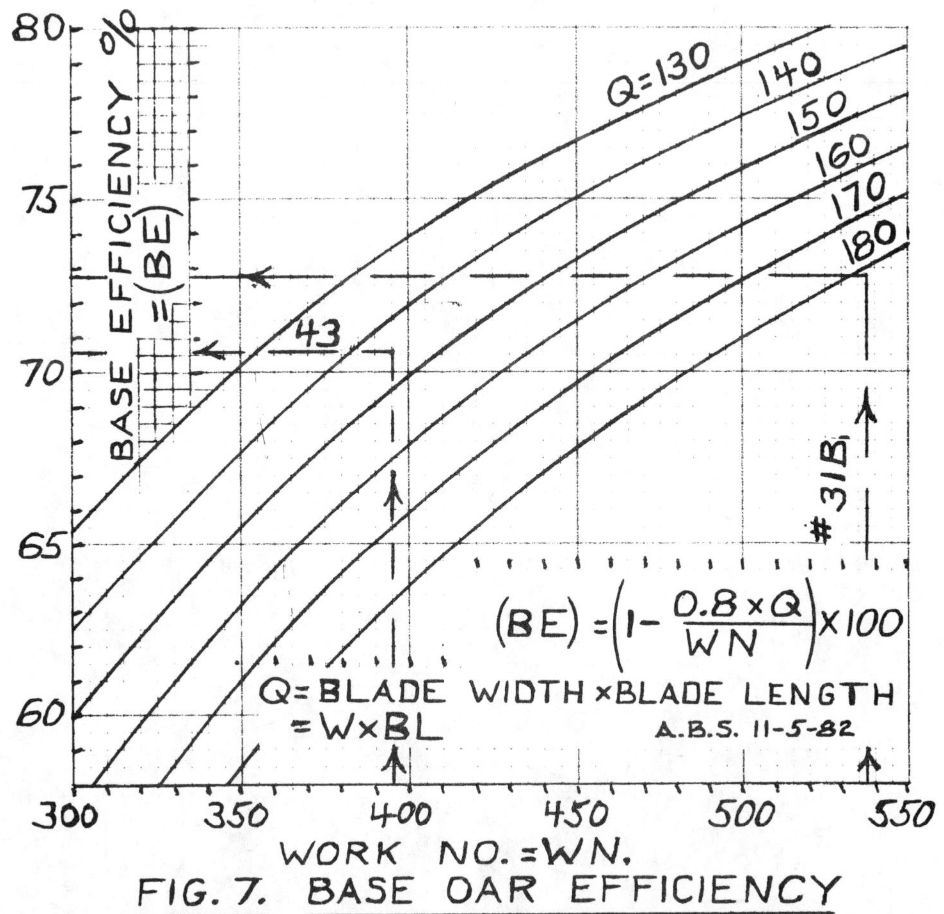

FIG. 7. BASE OAR EFFICIENCY

FIG. 10. OAR SELECTION CALCULATIONS

COL. 1	COL. 2. EXISTING ALL DUTY OAR	COL. 3 NEW DOWN-WIND OAR
DIMENSIONS:		
A = TOT. LENGTH. IN.	90.	** 101" = 8'-5"
B = INNER LOOM "	23.	* 25.5
BL = BLADE LENGTH "	26.	* 23.5
BL/5 "	5.2	* 4.7
W = BLADE WIDTH "	5.5	* 7.
BLADE AREA SQ. IN.	116	128
CALCULATIONS:		
A-B-BL IN.	41	52
A-B-BL/5 "	61.8	70.8
R = FORCE LEVER RATIO $= \frac{A-B-BL/5}{(B-2")}$	$\frac{61.8}{21}$ = 2.94	
PERFORMANCE:		
Y = R x W = PULL NO.	2.94 x 5.5 = 16.2	* 21
WN = Y (B-2") = WORK NO.	16.2 x 21 = 340	21 x 23.5 = 494
$(BE) = \frac{A-B-BL}{A-B-BL/5}$	$\frac{41.}{61.8}$ = 66%	$\frac{52}{70.8}$ 73%
BOAT:		
LOCK SPAN IN.	* 46	* 46
GRIP OVER LAP "	(2x23) - 46 = 0	(2x25.5) - 46 = 5
* ASSUMED		
** A = B + Y (B-2")/W + BL/5 =		25.5 + 70.5 + 4.7 = 101" = 8'-5"
		A.B.S 10-17-92

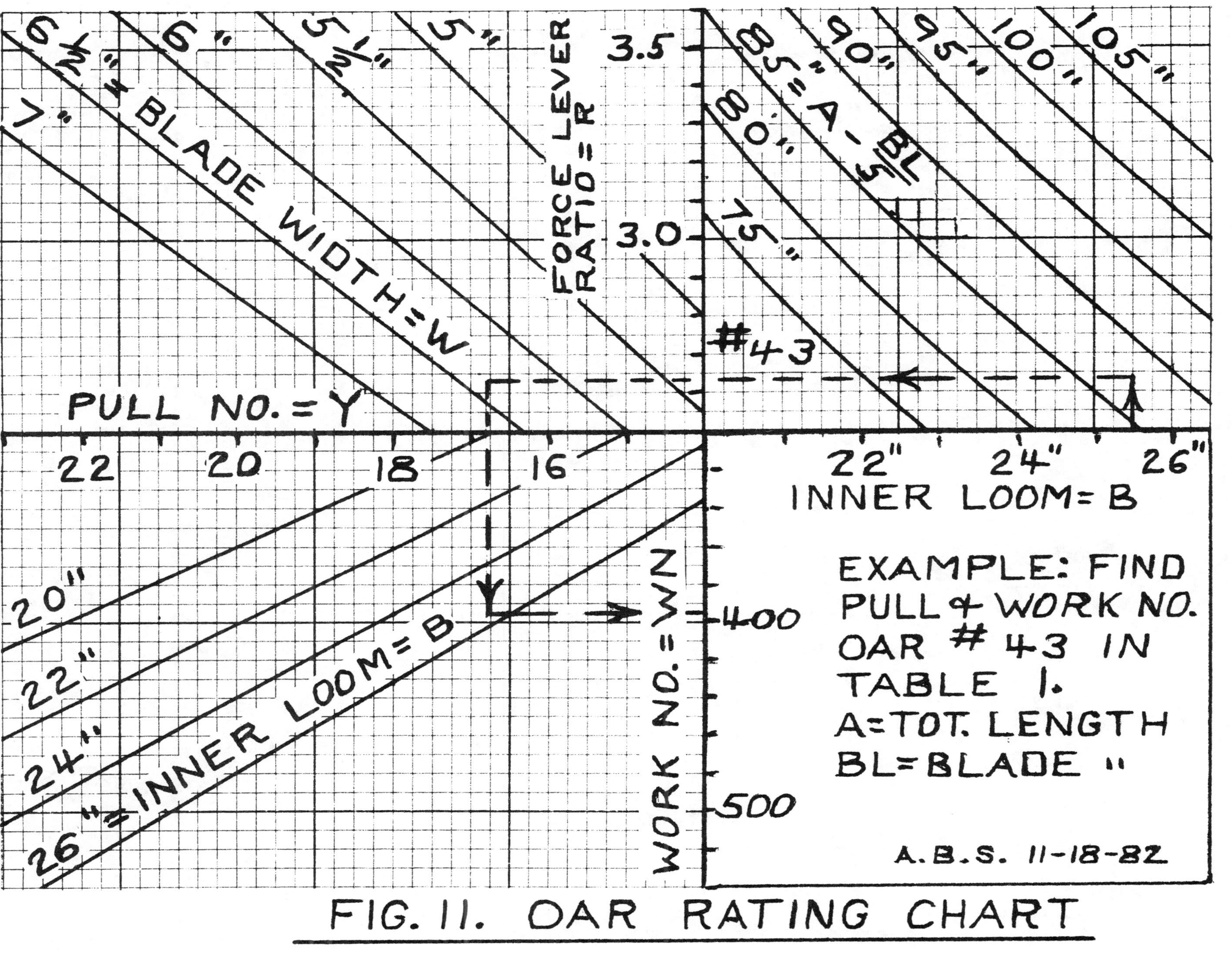

FIG. 11. OAR RATING CHART

FIG. 12. OAR SELECTION

SUGGESTED TRIAL PULL NUMBERS. Y

ADULTS IN GOOD SHAPE-	MALE	FEMALE
CALM & UP-WIND OARS	16.	15.

SHORT RACES - ADD 10%
LONG RACES - DEDUCT 10%

DOWN-WIND OARS	21.	19.

FOR A SURGING LIGHT BOAT ADD 5%.
RACING CRITERION FOR Y IS TO BE HIGH ENOUGH TO TEMPORARILY EXHAUST ROWER AT RACE'S END AT ABOUT 50 STROKES/MIN. FOR SHORT RACE AND LESS FOR LONG RACE. MAKE RACING WN HIGH.

DESIGN EQUATION FOR A NEW OAR.

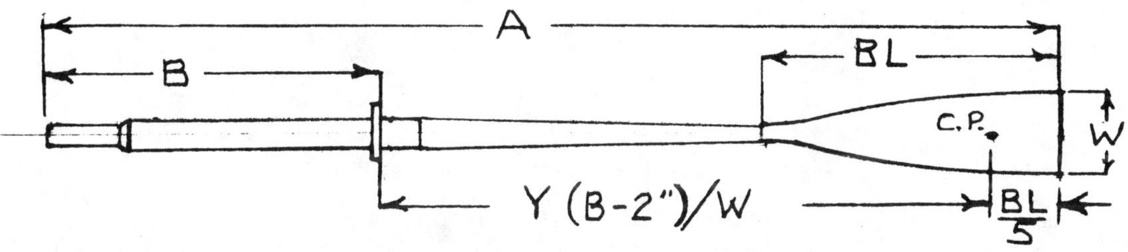

$$A = B + Y(B - 2")/W + BL/5$$

NOMENCLATURE IN TABLE 1.

A.B.S. 10-17-92.

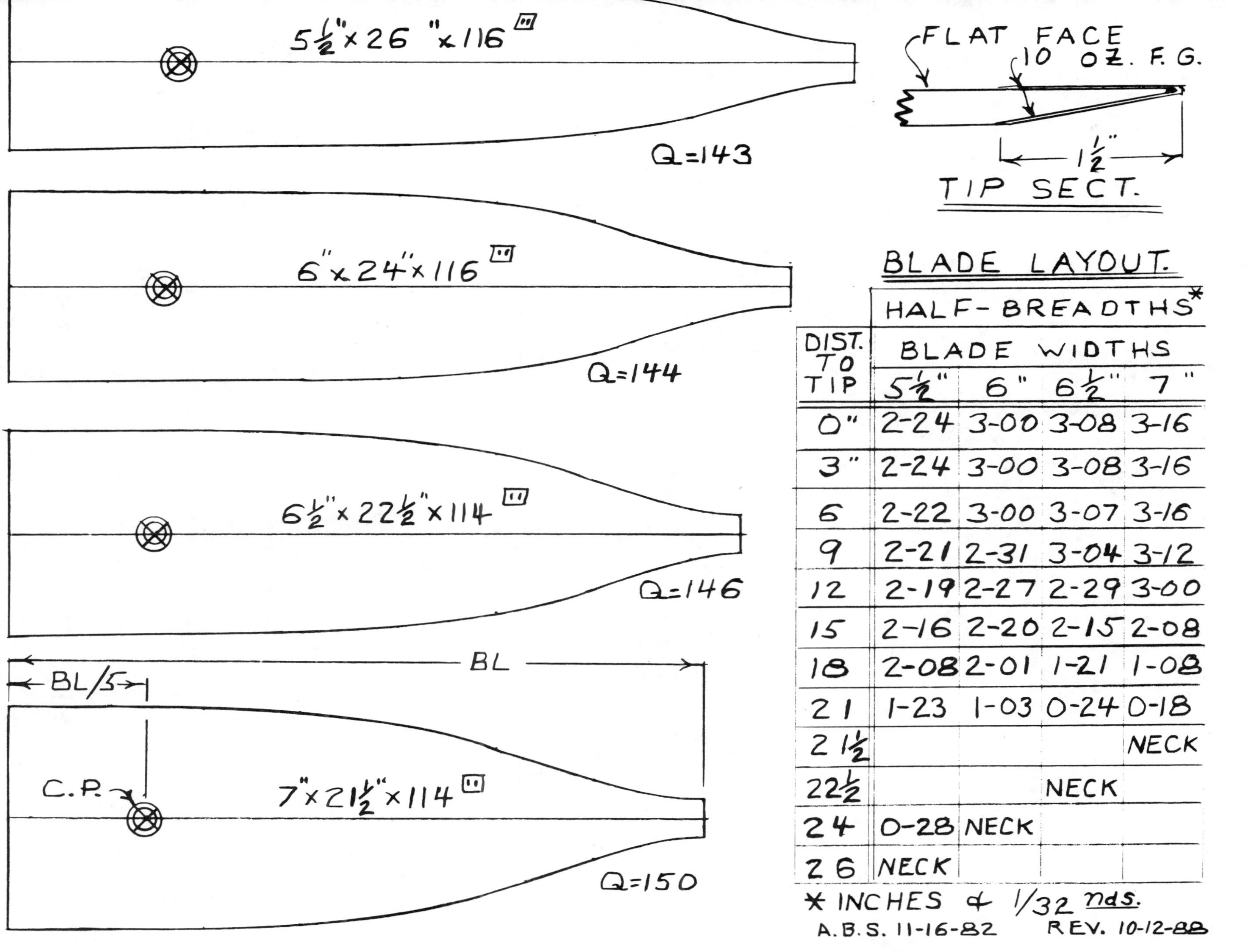

BLADE LAYOUT.

DIST. TO TIP	HALF-BREADTHS* BLADE WIDTHS 5½"	6"	6½"	7"
0"	2-24	3-00	3-08	3-16
3"	2-24	3-00	3-08	3-16
6	2-22	3-00	3-07	3-16
9	2-21	2-31	3-04	3-12
12	2-19	2-27	2-29	3-00
15	2-16	2-20	2-15	2-08
18	2-08	2-01	1-21	1-08
21	1-23	1-03	0-24	0-18
21½				NECK
22½			NECK	
24	0-28	NECK		
26	NECK			

* INCHES & 1/32 nds.

A.B.S. 11-16-82 REV. 10-12-88

FIG. 13. STRAIGHT BLADE SHAPES

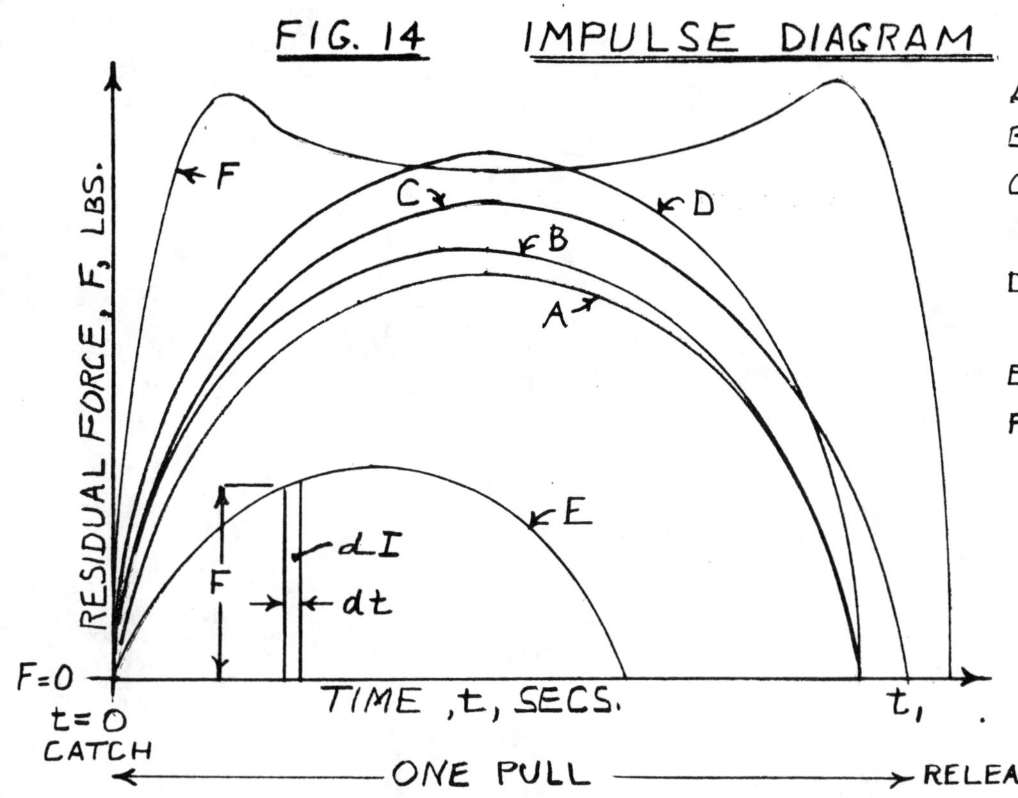

DERIVATION: NEWTON'S 2nd LAW; $F = ma$

CHANGE TO ENGLISH UNITS: $F = \frac{W}{g} \times a$

PUT IN DIFFERENTIAL FORM: $a = \frac{dV}{dt}$, SO $F = \frac{W}{g} \cdot \frac{dV}{dt}$

TRANSPOSE dt: $Fdt = \frac{W}{g} \cdot dV$ IMPULSE IS FORCE × TIME.

Fdt IS DIFFERENTIAL OF IMPULSE $dI = FdT$ WHICH IS AREA OF SLICE FROM TIME AXIS UP TO IMPULSE CURVE.

INTEGRATE: $$\int dI = \int_{t=t_0}^{t=t_1} Fdt = \frac{W}{g} \int_{V=V_0}^{V=V_1} dV = I$$

WT. OF BOAT AND CONTENTS AND LOCATION OF C.G. ASSUMED CONSTANT SO OUTSIDE OF INTEGRAL SIGN.

I = TOTAL AREA UNDER IMPULSE CURVE.

SO $\frac{W}{g}(V_1 - V_0) = I$

$\frac{W}{g} \cdot V_1$ = BOAT MOMENTUM AT END OF PULL.

$\frac{W}{g} \cdot V_0$ " " " CATCH.

$V_1 - V_0$ = CHANGE IN BOAT VEL., FT/SEC., DURING PULL.

NOTE: F = RESIDUAL FORWARD FORCE ON BOAT AT ANY INSTANT AFTER DEDUCTING RESISTANCE, LBS., OF HULL, WIND, AND CHOP FROM TOTAL FORWARD FORCE OF OARS.

FIG. 15 TRUE BLADE DIG ANGLE WITH CANTED LOCK

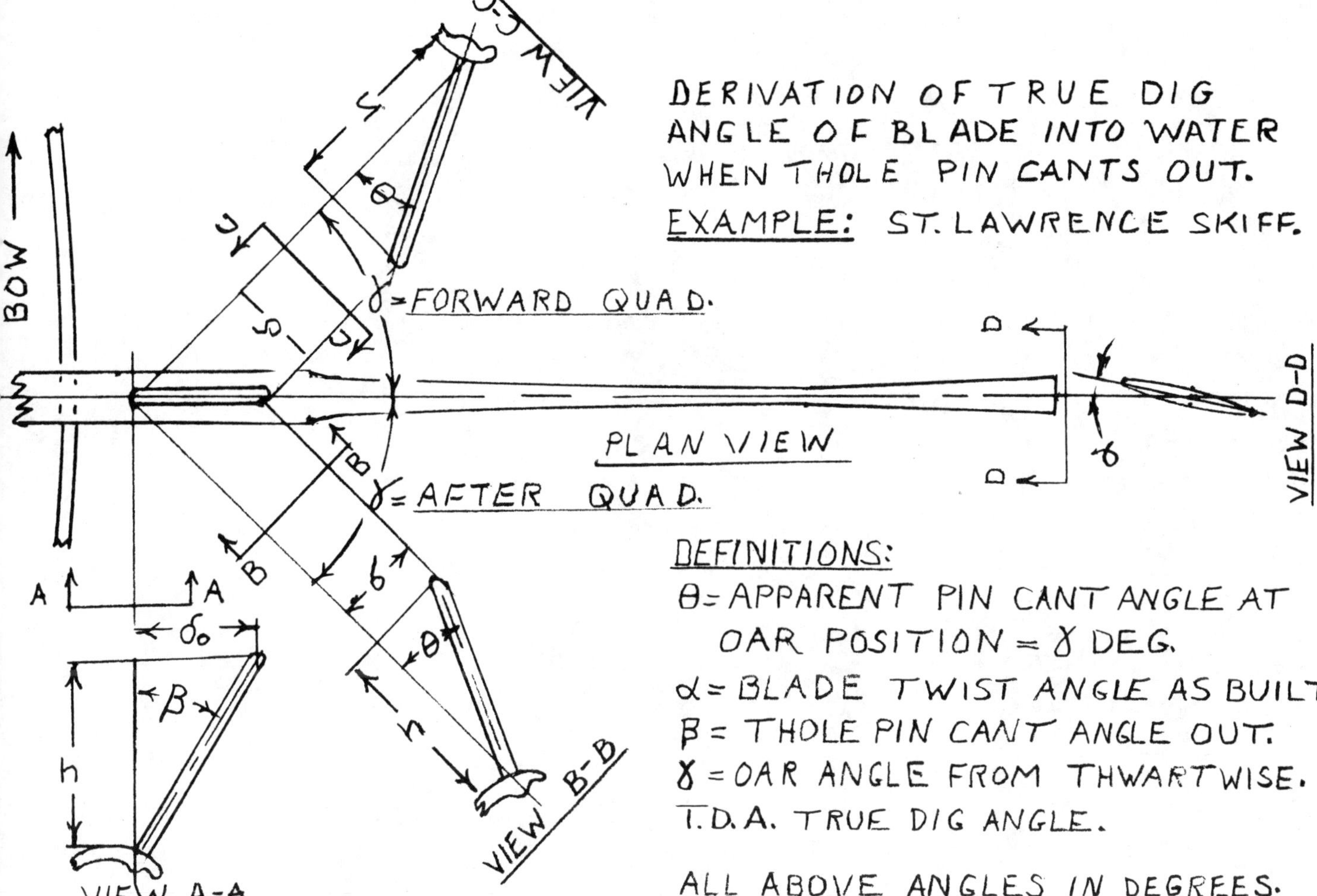

DEFINITIONS:

θ = APPARENT PIN CANT ANGLE AT OAR POSITION = γ DEG.

α = BLADE TWIST ANGLE AS BUILT.

β = THOLE PIN CANT ANGLE OUT.

γ = OAR ANGLE FROM THWARTWISE.

T.D.A. TRUE DIG ANGLE.

ALL ABOVE ANGLES IN DEGREES.

FORWARD QUADRANT $\delta = \delta_o \sin \gamma$

$$\frac{\delta}{h} = \tan \theta = \frac{\delta_o}{h} \sin \gamma = \tan \beta \cdot \sin \gamma$$

FOR SMALL ANGLES: $\tan \theta \cong \theta$, AND $\tan \beta \cong \beta$ (RADIANS)

SO IN DEGREES $\theta = \beta \sin \gamma$

∴ TRUE DIG ANGLE = T.D.A. = $\alpha - \theta = \alpha - \beta \sin \gamma$

AFTER QUADRANT

BY SIMILAR REASONING, T.D.A. = $\alpha + \theta = \alpha + \beta \sin \gamma$

CHECK: WHEN $\beta = 0$ DEG. FOR NO PIN CANT ANGLE, T.D.A. = α FOR ALL OAR POSITIONS.

WHEN PIN CANTS (OUTWARD / INWARD), DIG ANGLE (INCREASES / DECREASES) DURING PULL.

A.B.S. 11-15-91

FIG. 16.

ST. LAWRENCE SKIFF OAR LOCKS.

DETERMINATION OF TRUE BLADE DIG ANGLE INTO WATER WITH OUTWARD CANTED THOLE PIN.

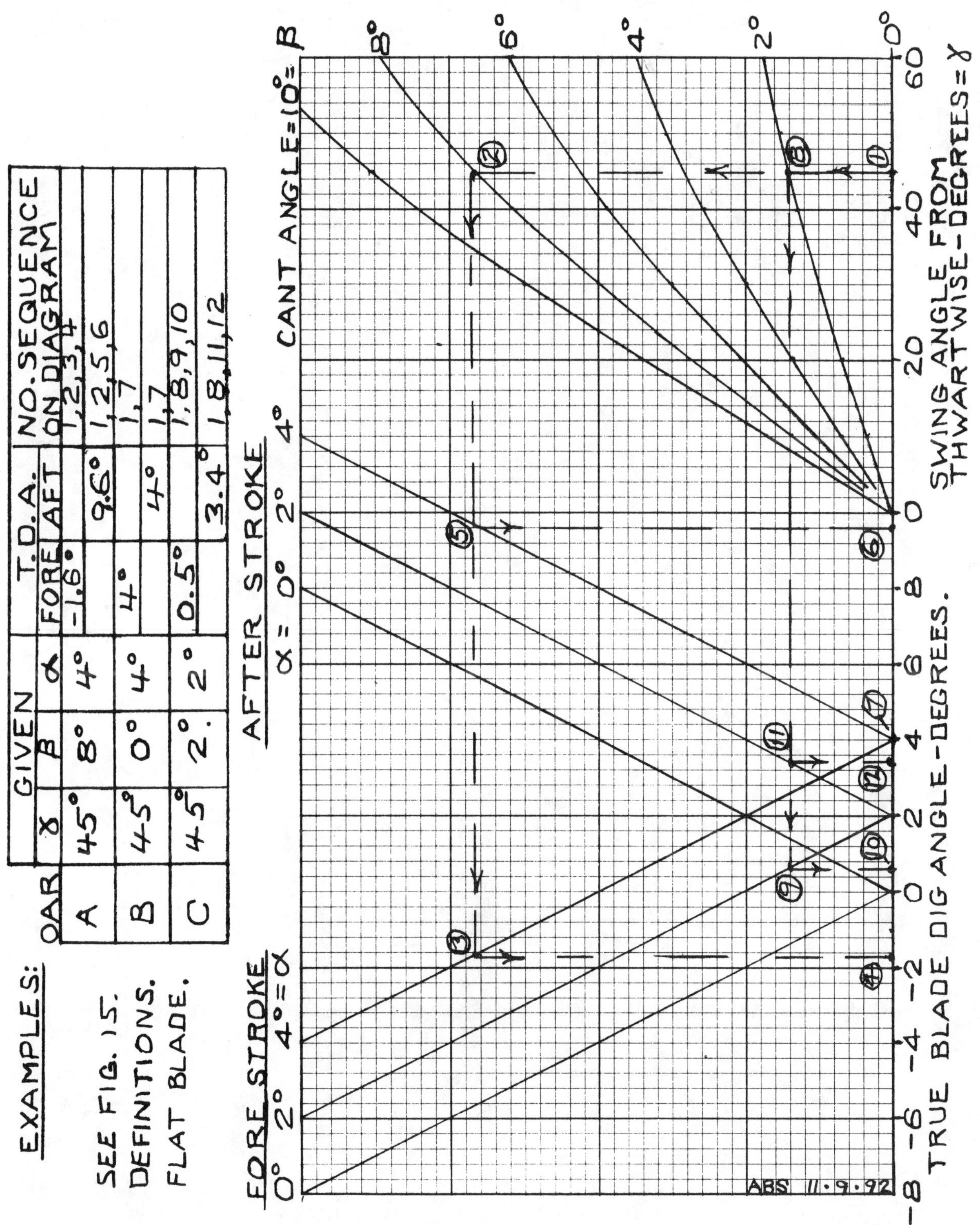

OAR	GIVEN γ	GIVEN β	GIVEN α	T.D.A. FORE	T.D.A. AFT	NO. SEQUENCE ON DIAGRAM
A	45°	8°	4°	-1.6°		1,2,3,4
					9.6°	1,2,5,6
B	45°	0°	4°	4°		1,7
					4°	1,7
C	45°	2°	2°	0.5°		1,8,9,10
					3.4°	1,8,11,12

FIG. 17 SOME IRISH CURRAGH OARS

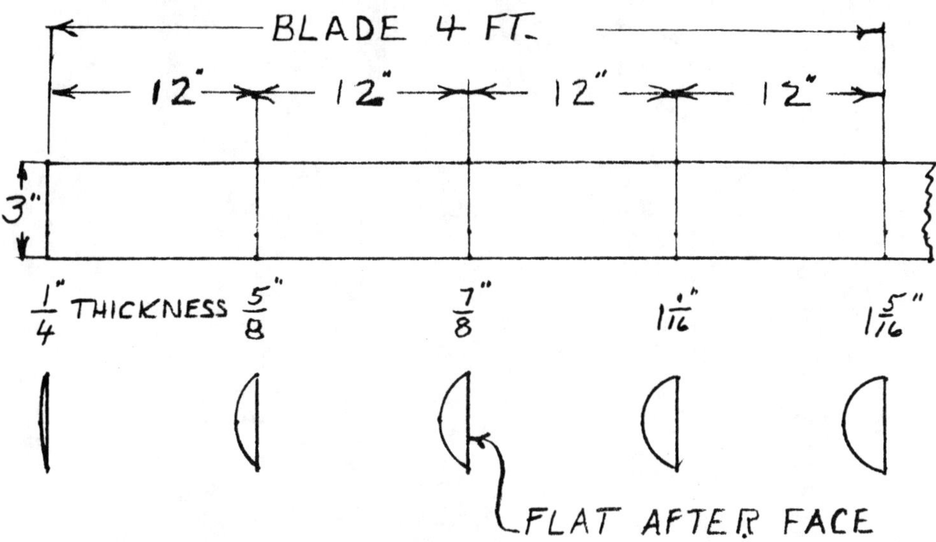

8 FT. LENGTH OVERALL.
23" INNER LOOM LENGTH
OAR IS VERY LIMBER.

23 FT. - 3 MAN - PLANKED - BOSTON CURRAGH.

COUNTY KERRY OARS *

11 FT. LENGTH
BLADE $2\frac{1}{4}$" WIDE, TAPERED TO $\frac{1}{2}$" TH. FLAT BOTH SIDES.

ARAN ISLS OARS*

10 FT. LONG.

* REF. HORNELL, J., "THE CURRAGHS OF IRELAND," MARINERS MIRROR VOL XXIV #1 JAN. 1938, JOURNAL OF SOC'Y FOR NAUTICAL RES., CAMBRIDGE UNIV. PRESS.

A.B.S. 11-16-91

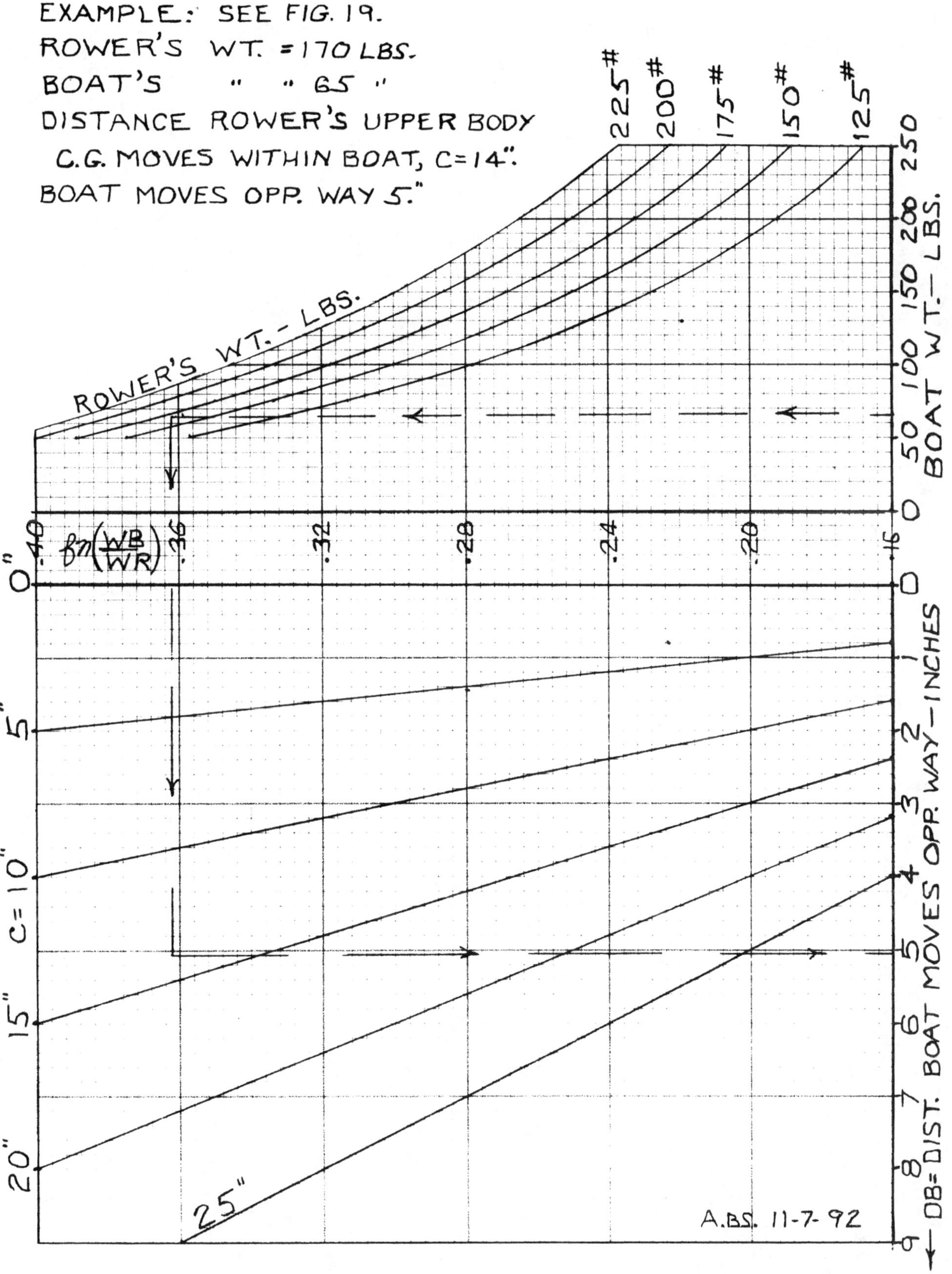
FIG. 18
MOMENTUM DIAGRAM — FIXED SEAT ROWBOAT
EXAMPLE: SEE FIG. 19.
ROWER'S WT. = 170 LBS.
BOAT'S " " 65 "
DISTANCE ROWER'S UPPER BODY C.G. MOVES WITHIN BOAT, C=14".
BOAT MOVES OPP. WAY 5."
225#
200#
175#
150#
125#
ROWER'S WT. - LBS.
BOAT WT. - LBS.
0
50
100
150
200
250
.40
.36
.32
.28
.24
.20
.16
fn(WB/WR)
0"
5"
C=10"
15"
20"
25"
DB=DIST. BOAT MOVES OPP. WAY—INCHES
0
1
2
3
4
5
6
7
8
9
A.BS. 11-7-92

FIG. 19 FIXED SEAT.

DERIVATION OF MOMENTUM EQUATIONS AND GRAPH.

ASSUME BOAT AND OARS MOTIONLESS AT START, OARS OUT OF WATER.
COMBINED C.G. ROWER AND BOAT AT PT. (5). SEE BELOW,
DOESN'T MOVE WHEN APPLYING LAW OF CONS. MOMENTUM.
WR = ROWER'S WT. WITH C.G. INITIALLY AT PT. (1).
WB = BOAT'S " " " " " PT. (3).
ROWER MOVES FORWARD, PT. (1) TO PT. (2). BOAT AFT, PT. (3) TO (4).
VR = ROWER'S FORWARD VELOCITY WITH RESPECT TO PT. (5).
VB = BOATS VELOCITY ASTERN " " " " ".
BY CONS. OF MOM. $\overleftarrow{WR \times VR} = \overrightarrow{WB \times VB}$. — — — — (A)
TIME TO GO (1) TO (2) EQUALS (3) TO (4). DIST. = TIME x VEL.
THEN DIST. DR (1) TO (2) IS PROP'NL TO VEL. VR FROM (1) TO (2).
AND " DB (3) " (4) " " " " VB " (3) " (4).
SO CONS. LAW (A) CAN BE WRITTEN $\overleftarrow{WR \times DR} = \overrightarrow{WB \times DB}$
OR DB = DR(WR/WB) —— —— —— —— (B)
HOWEVER, TOTAL DIST. FORWARD THE ROWER MOVES IN
THE BOAT WITH RESPECT TO BOAT'S C.G. = DR + DB.
LET DR + DB = C WHICH CAN BE ESTIMATED FROM TOT.
MOVEMENT FORWARD OF ROWER'S UPPER BODY C.G. - - - - (C)
SUBSTITUTE (C) IN (B): DB = (C − DB)(WR/WB)

DIST. BOAT GOES = DB = $\dfrac{C}{\left(\dfrac{WB}{WR} + 1\right)}$.

EXAMPLE FIXED SEAT

FOR 170 LB. ROWER, WR = 170/2 = 85 LBS.
65 " BOAT, WB = 65 + 85 = 150.
TOT. 235 " TOT. 235 "
WB/WR = 1.76; (WB/WR) + 1 = 2.76
EST. MOVEMENT ROWER'S UPPER
BODY C.G. = 14" FORWARD.
DIST. BOAT MOVES AFT = DB = 14/2.76 = 5"

A.B.S. 11·3·92

Bibliography

There are some good English references on rowing which are rather technical and directed to sliding-seat racing. However, there is something to be learned from them relevant to pleasure rowing if one is willing to dig diligently. Some of these references are hard to find. Not all of them agree with the present article on oar design. I will let the reader figure out what to believe in this ancient and fascinating field.

Alexander, F.H. "The propulsive Efficiency of Rowing." Transactions of the Institution of Naval Architects (July 1927).

Bolger, Philip C. "On Rowing." Yachting (April 1975).

Bourne, G.C. Text Book of Oarsmanship. Oxford: Oxford University Press, 1925.

Culler, Robert D. Boats, Oars, and Rowing. Camden, Maine: International Marine Publishing, 1978.

Durham, W., Mariner's Catalogue, Volume 4. Camden, Maine: International Marine Publishing, 1976.

Edwards, H.R.A. The Way of a Man with a Blade. London: Routledge & Kegan Paul, 1963.

Gardner, John. National Fisherman (April 1972).

_______. National Fisherman (February, March, April, May 1980).

_______. in Durant, Kenneth and Helen. The Adirondack Guide Boat. Camden, Maine: International Marine Publishing, 1980.

Glendon, R.A. and R.J. Rowing. Philadelphia: J.B. Lippincott, 1923.

Hornell, J. "The Curraghs of Ireland." Mariner's Mirror 24 (January 1938).

Lethbridge, T.C., Boats and Boatmen. London: Thames and Hudson, 1952.

Marchaj, C.A., *Aero-Hydrodynamics of Sailing*. New York: Dodd, Mead, 1979.

Martin, D. *WoodenBoat* 48 (September/October 1982): 54.

M.I.N.A. "The Mechanics of English & Belgian Rowing." *The Yachting & Boating Monthly* (September 1907): 381-84.

Simmons, W.J. *Small Boat Journal* (November 1982): 58-61.

Steever, Andrew B. "Howard Seaman and the Adirondack Racing Guide Boat." Manuscript and movies 1988, Adirondack Museum, Blue Mountain Lake, New York.

Stensgaard, G.N. *Lines & Offsets* 21 (December 1979), 30 (October 1981).

Taylor, Roger. *WoodenBoat* 42 (September/October 1981): 39.

van der Waerden, R. "The Theory and Practice of Belgian Rowing." *The Yachting & Boating Monthly* (January 1908): 209-12.

Washington Post, 29 April 1990, B-14.

Webb, P.H. "Form and Function in Fish Swimming." *Scientific American* (July 1984).

Williams, J.G.P., and Scott, A.C. *Rowing: A Scientific Approach*. New York: A.S. Barnes & Co., 1967.

Wilson, P.C. *Modern Rowing*. Harrisburg, Pennsylvania: Stackpole Books, 1969.

WoodenBoat 18 (September/October 1977): 57.